Left Ventricular Assist Devices

Guest Editors

JOHN A. ELEFTERIADES, MD
DONALD M. BOTTA Jr, MD

CARDIOLOGY CLINICS

www.cardiology.theclinics.com

Consulting Editor
MICHAEL H. CRAWFORD, MD

November 2011 • Volume 29 • Number 4

SAUNDERS an imprint of ELSEVIER, Inc.

W.B. SAUNDERS COMPANY
A Division of Elsevier Inc.

1600 John F. Kennedy Blvd. • Suite 1800 • Philadelphia, PA 19103-2899

http://www.theclinics.com

CARDIOLOGY CLINICS Volume 29, Number 4
November 2011 ISSN 0733-8651, ISBN-13: 978-1-4557-1026-3

Editor: Barbara Cohen-Kligerman
Developmental Editor: Teia Stone

Cardiology Clinics (ISSN 0733-8651) is published quarterly by Elsevier Inc., 360 Park Avenue South, New York, NY 10010-1710. Months of issue are February, May, August, and November. Business and Editorial Offices: 1600 John F. Kennedy Blvd., Ste. 1800, Philadelphia, PA 19103-2899. Customer Service Office: 3251 Riverport Lane, Maryland Heights, MO 63043. Periodicals postage paid at New York, NY and additional mailing offices. Subscription prices are $282.00 per year for US individuals, $458.00 per year for US institutions, $139.00 per year for US students and residents, $345.00 per year for Canadian individuals, $569.00 per year for Canadian institutions, $400.00 per year for international individuals, $569.00 per year for international institutions and $196.00 per year for Canadian and international students/residents. To receive student/resident rate, orders must be accompanied by name of affiliated institution, data of term, and the *signature* of program/residency coordinator on institution letterhead. Orders will be billed at individual rate until proof of status is received. Foreign air speed delivery is included in all *Clinics* subscription prices. All prices are subject to change without notice. **POSTMASTER:** Send address changes to *Cardiology Clinics*, Elsevier Health Sciences Division, Subscription Customer Service, 3251 Riverport Lane, Maryland Heights, MO 63043. **Customer Service: 1-800-654-2452 (U.S. and Canada); 314-447-8871 (outside U.S. and Canada). Fax: 314-447-8029. E-mail: journalscustomerservice-usa@elsevier.com (for print support); journalsonlinesupport-usa@ elsevier.com (for online support).**

Reprints. For copies of 100 or more, of articles in this publication, please contact the Commercial Reprints Department, Elsevier Inc., 360 Park Avenue South, New York, NY 10010-1710. Tel.: 212-633-3812; Fax: 212-462-1935; E-mail: reprints@elsevier.com.

Cardiology Clinics is also published in Spanish by McGraw-Hill Interamericana Editores S. A., P.O. Box 5-237, 06500, Mexico D. F., Mexico; in Portuguese by Reichmann and Alfonso Editores Rio de Janeiro, Brazil; and in Greek by Dimitrios P. Lagos, 8 Pondon Street, GR115-28 Ilissia, Greece.

Cardiology Clinics is covered in *MEDLINE/PubMed (Index Medicus), Excerpta Medica, The Cumulative Index to Nursing and Allied Health Literature* (CINAHL).

Printed and bound by CPI Group (UK) Ltd, Croydon, CR0 4YY

Transferred to Digital Print 2011

Contributors

CONSULTING EDITOR

MICHAEL H. CRAWFORD, MD
Professor of Medicine, University of California, San Francisco; Lucie Stern Chair in Cardiology and Chief of Clinical Cardiology, University of California, San Francisco Medical Center, San Francisco, California

GUEST EDITORS

JOHN A. ELEFTERIADES, MD
William W.L. Glenn Professor of Surgery; Director, Aortic Institute at Yale-New Haven School of Medicine, New Haven, Connecticut

DONALD M. BOTTA Jr, MD
Cardiovascular Surgeons, P.A., Orlando, Florida

AUTHORS

OLTJAN ALBAJRAMI, MD
Department of Internal Medicine, St Mary's Hospital, Waterbury, Connecticut

CARLO R. BARTOLI, PhD
MD/PhD Program, Department of Physiology and Biophysics, University of Louisville School of Medicine, Louisville, Kentucky

LAVANYA BELLUMKONDA, MD
Instructor, Division of Cardiology, Department of Internal Medicine, Yale School of Medicine, New Haven, Connecticut

PRAMOD BONDE, MD
Director, Mechanical Circulatory Support, Section of Cardiac Surgery, Yale School of Medicine, New Haven, Connecticut

DONALD M. BOTTA Jr, MD
Cardiovascular Surgeons, P.A., Orlando, Florida

JOHN V. CONTE, MD
Associate Director of Cardiac Surgery, Division of Cardiac Surgery, Department of Surgery, Johns Hopkins Cardiac Surgery, The Johns Hopkins Medical Institutions, Baltimore, Maryland

ROBERT D. DOWLING, MD
Department of Surgery, University of Louisville, Louisville, Kentucky

JOHN A. ELEFTERIADES, MD
William W. L. Glenn Professor of Surgery; Director, Aortic Institute at Yale-New Haven School of Medicine, New Haven, Connecticut

MICHAEL IBRAHIM, BA (Cantab)
Heart Science Centre, Magdi Yacoub Institute, Harefield Hospital, London, United Kingdom

DANIEL JACOBY, MD
Assistant Professor of Medicine, Division of Cardiology, Department of Internal Medicine, Yale School of Medicine, New Haven, Connecticut

ROBERT JARVIK, MD
Jarvik Heart, Inc., New York, New York

DAVID J. KACZOROWSKI, MD
Fellow in Cardiovascular Surgery, Division
of Cardiovascular Surgery, University of
Pennsylvania, Philadelphia, Pennsylvania

ABEEL A. MANGI, MD
Division of Cardiac Surgery, Yale University
School of Medicine, New Haven, Connecticut

YOSHIFUMI NAKA, MD, PhD
Department of Surgery, Columbia University
Medical Center, New York, New York

DANIEL PEREDA, MD
Advanced Cardiac Surgery Fellow, Division
of Cardiac Surgery, Department of Surgery,
Johns Hopkins Cardiac Surgery, The Johns
Hopkins Medical Institutions, Baltimore,
Maryland

ALANSON SAMPLE, PhD
Department of Electrical Engineering,
University of Washington, Seattle, Washington

JOSHUA SMITH, PhD
Department of Electrical Engineering;
Department of Computer Science and
Engineering, University of Washington,
Seattle, Washington

LOUIS H. STEIN, MD
Section of Cardiac Surgery, Yale
University School of Medicine,
New Haven, Connecticut

HIROO TAKAYAMA, MD
Department of Surgery, Columbia University
Medical Center, New York, New York

BENJAMIN WATERS, BS
Department of Electrical Engineering,
University of Washington, Seattle,
Washington

Y. JOSEPH WOO, MD
Associate Professor of Surgery, Director
of Cardiac Transplantation and Mechanical
Circulatory Support Program, Division
of Cardiovascular Surgery, University
of Pennsylvania, Philadelphia, Pennsylvania

CESARE M. TERRACCIANO, MD, PhD
Heart Science Centre, Magdi Yacoub Institute,
Harefield Hospital, London, United Kingdom

JONATHAN A. YANG, MD
Department of Surgery, Columbia University
Medical Center, New York, New York

MAGDI H. YACOUB, FRS
Heart Science Centre, Magdi Yacoub
Institute, Harefield Hospital, London,
United Kingdom

Contents

> The pathophysiology of heart failure is complex, and downstream effects cause decline in multiple systems. Medical therapies intended to slow or reverse disease progression have been shown to improve prognosis in prospective trials. Improvement in prognosis has also been observed in large cohorts across time strata. However, near-term mortality for those with advanced disease remains unacceptably high. Prognosis in advanced heart failure may be assessed with the appropriate use of clinical prediction tools. Optimal timing of evaluation for heart transplantation and/or mechanical circulatory support depends on an understanding of these issues.

> Left ventricular assist device therapy as a destination therapy for end-stage heart failure has made a large leap with continuous flow devices. Continuous flow does not seem to have a detrimental effect on end-organ function, at least in the midterm. Various expected and unexpected complications have been reported associated with this technology. More experience and research are warranted.

> Left ventricular assist device (LVAD) placement is a serious surgical procedure. At our center, we accumulated a very large experience with the Novacor LVAD from the very first clinical trial, as well as from more recent experiences with the Jarvik 2000 and the HeartMate II. This article discusses technical issues that are common to all durable LVAD devices, with special emphasis on strategy and technical considerations aimed at avoiding surgical pitfalls.

which they function, and implications for patient management. This article discusses devices that are being developed or are in clinical trials. Devices are categorized as standard full support, less-invasive full support, partial support: rotary pumps, partial support: counterpulsation devices, right ventricular assist device, and total artificial heart. Implantation strategy, mechanism of action, durability, efficacy, hemocompatibility, and human factors are considered. The feasibility of novel strategies for unloading the failing heart is examined.

Transplant or VAD?   585

Robert Jarvik

Major advances in vascular assist device (VAD) technology and the clinical acceptance of destination therapy for patients with contraindications to transplant raise the questions of what patient benefit is necessary to recommend VAD implant for long-term support in patients who are transplant candidates. What are the appropriate indications for use and timing considerations for long-term VAD therapy in patients who qualify for transplant but are unlikely to obtain a donor? The authors suggest that VAD implantation for the indication of "maintenance therapy" where patients must remain on the VAD for two years before becoming transplant eligible, would constitute an appropriate clinical avenue to study these issues.

Who Needs an RVAD in Addition to an LVAD?   599

David J. Kaczorowski and Y. Joseph Woo

Mechanical circulatory support using left ventricular assist devices (LVAD) has become an accepted mode of therapy for both bridging patients with end-stage heart failure to transplant and as a destination therapy. Right ventricular (RV) dysfunction is common after LVAD insertion and is a significant source of morbidity and mortality in patients undergoing LVAD placement. Several studies have identified clinical, laboratory, hemodynamic, and echocardiographic parameters that may serve as risk factors for RV dysfunction after LVAD placement. Furthermore, scoring systems have been established to help quantitatively predict the potential need for RV support after LVAD placement.

Toward Total Implantability Using Free-Range Resonant Electrical Energy Delivery System: Achieving Untethered Ventricular Assist Device Operation Over Large Distances   609

Benjamin Waters, Alanson Sample, Joshua Smith, and Pramod Bonde

Heart failure is a terminal disease with a very poor prognosis. Although the gold standard of treatment remains heart transplant, only a minority of patients can benefit from transplants. Another promising alternative is mechanical circulatory assistance using ventricular assist devices. The authors envision a completely implantable cardiac assist system affording tether-free mobility in an unrestricted space powered

Cardiology Clinics

READ THE CLINICS ONLINE!
Access your subscription at:
www.theclinics.com

Foreword

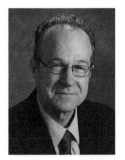

Michael H. Crawford, MD
Consulting Editor

The February 2003 issue of *Cardiology Clinics* was titled Ventricular Assist Devices and the Artificial Heart. At that time, using the early devices as a bridge to transplantation was fairly well accepted, but destination therapy with a mechanical device was highly controversial. Now, 8 years later, destination therapy is no longer as controversial. This is not because the newer devices have achieved long-term flawless performance, but rather because use of long-term mechanical assist devices has allowed a significant proportion of diseased hearts to recover, such that the device can be removed. The concept of bridge to recovery or transplantation has re-energized this field. Thus, I was delighted when Dr John Elefteriades agreed to guest edit an issue of *Cardiology Clinics* to update this important topic.

He has assembled a world-renowned group of authors, including senior luminaries in the field such as Robert Jarvik and Sir Magdi Yacoub, to discuss the indications, applications, and management of these devices. Thorny topics such as the indications for right ventricular assist devices,

preventing driveline infections, and how to decide between a device and transplantation are covered. Also, there are articles on technical issues that will be of interest to those managing these patients. Finally, Dr Elefteriades comments on each article with a mini-editorial. This is a practice seen most commonly in surgical journals that adds an interesting twist to this issue of the *Clinics*.

Since most of our patients are eventually going to die of pump failure, this outstanding issue will be of considerable interest to all who care for patients with heart disease.

Michael H. Crawford, MD
Division of Cardiology, Department of Medicine
University of California
San Francisco Medical Center
505 Parnassus Avenue, Box 0124
San Francisco, CA 94143-0124, USA

E-mail address:
crawfordm@medicine.ucsf.edu

Cardiol Clin 29 (2011) xi
doi:10.1016/j.ccl.2011.09.002
0733-8651/11/$ – see front matter

cardiology.theclinics.com

Foreword

Preface
Left Ventricular Assist Devices

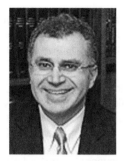 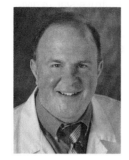

John A. Elefteriades, MD   Donald M. Botta Jr, MD
Guest Editors

In the current issue of *Cardiology Clinics*, a distinguished panel of authors examines and dissects important contemporary, and often controversial, topics in the treatment of advanced heart failure by mechanical assist devices.

We start with a frank assessment by Dr Jacoby and colleagues of whether advanced mechanical technology has truly produced improvement in the prognosis of heart failure—above and beyond the natural outlook as represented in the classic survival graph published by Franciosa and Cohn several decades ago. The authors provide evidence that substantial progress has indeed been made.

Dr Naka and colleagues describe for us the up-to-date armamentarium of devices currently available for "destination" therapy. They elaborate the benefits and liabilities of specific clinically approved assist devices.

Dr Botta and I address technical pitfalls common to surgical placement of various mechanical assist devices—pitfalls that can make literally a life and death difference in early and late patient outcome.

Driveline infections continue to be the Achilles' heel of mechanical left ventricular support. Many authorities believe that an infection is eventually inevitable whenever a driveline traverses the integument. Dr Conte and his colleague Dr Pereda examine the issue of driveline infection in detail, elucidating its high prevalence and its virulent adverse impact on patient outcome. They provide valuable advice on prevention and treatment of driveline infection.

Professor Sir Magdi Yacoub has pioneered the concept of mechanical bridge to recovery for advanced heart failure. He and his colleagues provide their current thoughts on this encouraging possible outcome of mechanical cardiac assistance—including guidance on how to promote and encourage recovery of the native heart.

I have asked Dr Naka and colleagues to address and compare specifics of the actual clinical use of currently available assist devices, each of which has important idiosyncrasies that bear careful study in order to achieve optimal outcome.

Mechanical left ventricular support is highly technological by its very nature. Technology tends to advance, and Dr Dowling and his colleague Dr Bartoli provide a thrilling glimpse into novel devices on the immediate horizon.

Dr Robert Jarvik, the brilliant mastermind of the field of mechanical cardiac assistance, electrified the world with the replacement of the native heart of Barney Clark by a mechanical device on December 2, 1982. I have asked him to discuss whether, if one of us required cardiac replacement, we would prefer a modern mechanical assist device or a heart transplant. Not surprisingly, Dr Jarvik points out multiple advantages and securities of mechanical assistance over and above certain intrinsic vagaries of transplantation. Which would you chose: device or transplant? Read this insightful article and re-assess.

One of the most difficult questions in mechanical cardiac assistance has to do with whether or not to supplement a mechanical left ventricular assist device (LVAD) with a right-sided device as well. The right ventricle can struggle or fail if left on its

Cardiol Clin 29 (2011) xiii–xiv
doi:10.1016/j.ccl.2011.09.001

own after LVAD placement. However, placement of a concomitant right ventricular device adds to the complexity of surgery and postoperative patient management. Dr Woo and Dr Kaczorowski provide objective data to guide us through this difficult decision-making.

Many authorities are of the opinion that, as long as a driveline pierces the integument, all mechanical devices will eventually become infected, if they remain in place long enough. Dr Bonde and colleagues describe an exciting experimental system that does not require any driveline that goes across the skin. Such systems represent the ultimate solution to the vexing problem of driveline and device infection. Dr Mangi gives us advice on how to predict, prevent, and treat right ventricular failure in LVAD recipients.

Dr Stein and I finish the issue. It is becoming increasingly appreciated that the nonpulsatile flow of current miniaturized axial flow LVADs leads to regressive changes in the arterial wall—changes that play a role in the colonic bleeding from arteriovenous malformations not uncommonly seen in LVAD patients. We propose, at the risk of controversy, that this ability of nonpulsatile flow to produce regression of the arterial wall to a more vein-like thinness might provide a tool useful in slowing or reversing rampant arteriosclerosis.

Each article is followed by a commentary by the editors highlighting key points made by each group of authors—as well as pointing out the strengths and weaknesses of the arguments made on these controversial, evolving topics.

We hope that the materials in this issue are of academic interest and clinical utility for both cardiologists and surgeons and their respective teams.

John A. Elefteriades, MD
Section of Cardiac Surgery
Yale University School of Medicine
Boardman 2
333 Cedar Street
New Haven, CT 06510, USA

Donald M. Botta Jr, MD
Cardiovascular Surgeons, P.A.
217 Hillcrest Street
Orlando, FL 32801, USA

E-mail addresses:
john.elefteriades@yale.edu (J.A. Elefteriades)
donald.botta@yale.edu (D.M. Botta Jr)

Natural History of End-stage LV Dysfunction: Has It Improved from the Classic Franciosa and Cohn Graph?

Daniel Jacoby, MD[a],*, Oltjan Albajrami, MD[b], Lavanya Bellumkonda, MD[a]

KEYWORDS
- Heart failure • Prognosis • Heart transplant
- Mechanical circulatory support

INCIDENCE, PREVALENCE, AND FINANCIAL IMPACT OF HEART FAILURE

Heart failure is a leading cause of hospitalization in the United States and, in 2010, accounted for 39 billion dollars in health care spending. The mortality is high after initial diagnosis, with 1 in 5 dying by year's end.[1] In the past 40 years, advances in medical and surgical therapies for heart failure have significantly improved the natural history of the disease. These therapies have arisen from, and been the nidus for, deeper understanding of the pathogenesis of disease and disease progression. Despite this, heart failure remains a chronic disease subject to time-dependent deterioration.[2] The advent of improved therapies has increased the prevalence and visibility of those suffering with advanced heart failure. Although arrival at this stage of disease is delayed, the prognosis once there is grave. Application of medical therapy at this stage of disease is fraught with failures, and application of surgical therapy (particularly heart transplant and mechanical circulatory support with left ventricular assist devices [LVADs] or biventricular assist devices [BiVADs]) may be limited by the onset of life-limiting end-organ

damage. Perhaps one of the side effects of the effective medical therapy now available for advanced heart failure is the ability to manage patients beyond the stage at which therapies such as heart transplantation or LVAD implantation are reasonable or practical. To highlight these issues, this article focuses on the major pathophysiologic mechanisms of heart failure, the most effective improvements in heart failure morbidity and mortality offered by medical therapy in the last 30 years, and prognostication in patients with advanced heart failure.

GRADING OF HEART FAILURE SEVERITY

One of the challenges of treating advanced heart failure is recognition of heart failure severity. Subjective assessment of heart failure class is limited by patient reporting, which is subject to patient expectation and self-assessment. For example, patients with social hesitancies (D-type personality) have been shown to underreport symptoms.[3] Objective measures of cardiac fitness and heart failure severity may be relied on in such cases to estimate both severity of symptoms

The authors have nothing to disclose.
[a] Division of Cardiology, Department of Internal Medicine, Yale School of Medicine, 367 Cedar Street, New Haven, CT 06519, USA
[b] Department of Internal Medicine, St Mary's Hospital, 56 Franklin Street, Waterbury, CT 06706, USA
* Corresponding author.
E-mail address: daniel.jacoby@yale.edu

Cardiol Clin 29 (2011) 485–495
doi:10.1016/j.ccl.2011.08.012

(metabolic exercise testing) and prognosis (Heart Failure Survival Score, Seattle Heart Failure Model).[4–7] However, despite agreement among heart failure experts on the usefulness of these assessments they are not routinely used by general cardiologists who follow most patients with advanced heart failure.

Heart failure class is commonly relied on to assess clinical status. New York Heart Association (NYHA) class predicts prognosis, as shown by outcomes among placebo groups from trials evaluating the efficacy of enalapril in treating heart failure with variable symptom severity.[8–10] However, heart failure class represents a moving target in any given patient. For example, patients may present with class 4 symptoms during initial and recurrent heart failure exacerbations. (See **Table 1**–NYHA Function Classification.) However, treatment, sometimes requiring the use of temporary mechanical support (intra-aortic balloon pump, catheter-based nonpulsatile assist devices) or continuous intravenous inotrope infusion, may lead to recompensation with resulting NYHA class 1 to 3 heart failure symptoms and the ability to discharge the patient on oral therapy. Classification of patients by heart failure stage does not suffer from the same variability. Heart failure stage was introduced to assist in standardization of application of therapies to those with heart failure (**Fig. 1**).

PATHOPHYSIOLOGY OF HEART FAILURE

Although there are exceptions, heart failure is generally viewed as a relentlessly progressive process. The early phases of disease are frequently asymptomatic but may also be associated with hemodynamic collapse, as in acute myocardial infarction and fulminant myocarditis. Although a waxing and waning clinical course is often seen, once the initial insult has occurred, ongoing decline is the general rule. Adverse cardiac remodeling, induced by intrinsic stressors, and the downstream effects of compensatory mechanisms combine to establish a cycle of repetitive

injury (**Fig. 2**).[11] Increased sympathetic tone,[12] activation of circulating and cardiac intrinsic neurohumoral factors, oxidative stress,[13] breakdown in myofibril calcium homeostasis,[14] programmed cell death,[15] upregulation of fibrosis,[16] and reduced efficiency of cardiac energetics all play a role in heart failure progression.[17] Failure of skeletal muscle, malnutrition, emotional stress, and comorbid disease are important cofactors in symptom expression and severity and also may play a role in the downward spiral of heart failure.[18–21]

THE SYMPATHETIC NERVOUS SYSTEM

Activation of the sympathetic nervous system is the initial physiologic response to an index event in heart failure. The clinical manifestations of increased sympathetic tone are increased resting heart rate, slowed heart rate recovery after exercise, and decreased heart rate variability.[22] Increased systemic vascular resistance, increased sodium retention, activation of the renal-angiotensin-aldosterone system, and increased circulating norepinephrine levels drive downstream volume retention, arrhythmogenesis, and adverse cardiac remodeling.[23]

THE RENAL-ANGIOTENSIN-ALDOSTERONE SYSTEM

Activation of the renal-angiotensin-aldosterone system is triggered both centrally and peripherally. Increased efferent norepinephrine and epinephrine directly increase renin secretion from the kidney. Meanwhile, reduced perfusion pressures at the afferent arteriole additionally stimulate renin release. Concentrations of both circulating and tissue-specific angiotensin-converting enzyme are increased, leading to exuberant angiotensin II activity. This potent vasoconstrictor maintains blood pressure at the expense of myocardial energy demands and also directly affects the myofibrils, with resulting hypertrophy and fibrosis.[16] Downstream release of aldosterone augments sodium and water retention and promotes myocyte hypertrophy as well as fibrosis.[24] These effects are adaptive in the setting of acute or decompensated heart failure, allowing for increased filling and contractility via the Frank-Starling mechanism, and for sustained perfusion to core systems. However, in intermediate and long-range time periods, these effects are predominantly maladaptive, leading to progressive cardiac dysfunction, inadequate organ perfusion, arrhythmias, and edema (both pulmonary and peripheral).

Table 1		
NYHA functional classification		
Class	**Definition**	
1	Asymptomatic	
2	Symptoms with moderate exertion	
3	Symptoms interfering with daily activities	
4	Symptoms at rest	

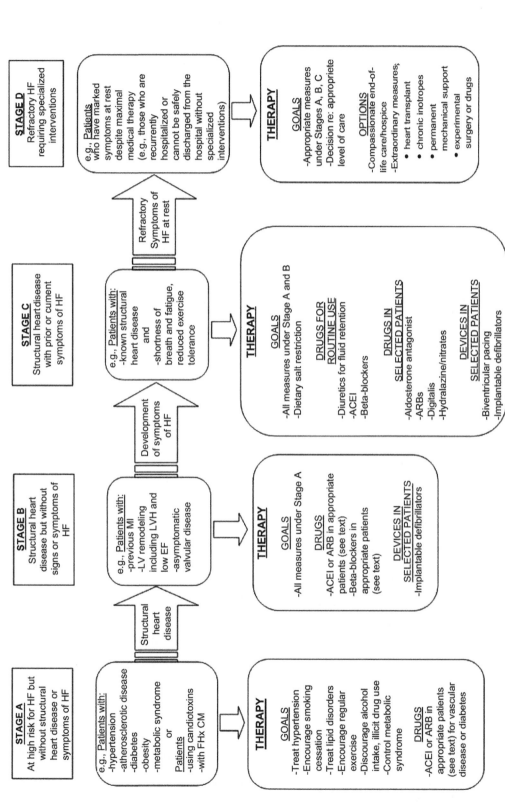

Fig. 1. Stages in the development of heart failure/recommended therapy by stage. ACEI, angiotensin-converting enzyme inhibitor; ARB, angiotensin II receptor blocker; EF, ejection fraction; FHx CM, family history of cardiomyopathy; HF, heart failure; LV, left ventricular; LVH, left ventricular hypertrophy; MI, myocardial infarction. (*From* Hunt SA, Abraham WT, Chin MH, et al. 2009 focused update incorporated into the ACC/AHA 2005 guidelines for the diagnosis and management of heart failure in adults. Circulation 2009;119:e398; with permission.)

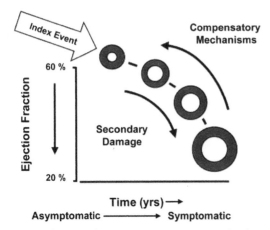

Fig. 2. After an index event, compensatory mechanisms initially compensate for acute dysfunction but, with chronic activation, contribute to secondary damage and both mechanical and clinical decompensation. (*From* Mann D, Bristow M. Mechanisms and models in heart failure: the biomechanical model and beyond. Circulation 2005;111:2838; with permission.)

OTHER PROCESSES

Apoptosis and autophagia seem to play a prominent role in adverse cardiac remodeling and fibrosis.[25] The triggers for these events are multifactorial and are still being investigated. Oxidative stress, adrenergic stimulation, and dysregulation of cardiac energetics play roles.[26,27] Hemodynamic stress plays a role in myocyte failure triggered via direct mechanical stress as well as via neurohumoral, paracrine, and endocrine pathways.[28] Clinical observation reveals that hemodynamic decompensation begets both progressive cardiac and visceral end-organ dysfunction as well as arrhythmogenesis, whereas restitution of hemodynamics provides an opportunity for cardiac and visceral organ recovery. These relationships strongly indicate that adverse hemodynamics are a central trigger for initiation and progression of maladaptive physiology. Acute and chronic heart failure represent hypercatabolic states.[29] Increased energy requirements in heart failure often overlap with decreased ability to ingest calories related to visceral congestion and malperfusion, leading to wasting and malnutrition.

Many of these effects are clinically observable with the use of commonly obtained clinical variables and laboratory values. Degrees of activation of these adaptive and maladaptive mechanisms correlate, sometimes loosely, sometimes closely, with prognosis in patients with heart failure. Therapies shown to improve survival in heart failure target the systems discussed earlier and lend credence to the neuroendocrine model of heart failure.

MEDICAL HEART FAILURE MEDICAL MANAGEMENT THAT IMPROVES PROGNOSIS
History of Heart Failure Therapy

In the early 1970s, Drs Franciosa and Cohn showed acute improvement in hemodynamics, exercise capacity, and metabolic effects with vasodilation using nitroprusside, hydralazine, and isosorbide dinitrate in patients with advanced left ventricular (LV) systolic failure.[30–32] The importance of neurohumoral regulation was further elucidated in the late 1970s with description of the role of sympathetic nervous system, renin-angiotensin system, and antidiuretic hormone, resulting in increased norepinephrine levels and hyponatremia.[33] Several clinical trials followed, testing inhibition using angiotensin-converting enzyme inhibitors (ACEIs), angiotensin receptor blockers (ARBs), aldosterone receptor antagonists and β-blockers to sequentially counter neurohumoral activation, resulting in significant improvements in morbidity and mortality.

ACEIs

Although afterload reduction is the ostensible mechanism of action of ACEIs, multiple downstream pathogenic processes have been implicated as mediators of ACEI benefit.[34–36] The CONSENSUS (Cooperative North Scandinavian Enalapril Survival Study) Trial, published in 1987, enrolled 253 patients with class 4 heart failure. Risk of death was 52% in the placebo group versus 36% in the treatment group, yielding a relative risk reduction of 30%.[10] Subsequent studies in patients with both milder heart failure symptoms and asymptomatic LV dysfunction have shown clinically and statistically significant reductions in mortality.[8,9] Reduction in mortality was attributable to reduction in heart failure deaths rather than arrhythmic death. In addition, use of ACEIs was associated with reduced ventricular size, increased left ventricular ejection fraction (LVEF), and improvement in heart failure symptoms. For patients intolerant of ACEIs, ARBs may prove similarly beneficial.[37,38] The potential additive effects of ACE/ARB therapy together remain controversial.

Nitrates and Hydralazine

This therapy was first tested in the V-HeFT trial, in which 642 patients with systolic dysfunction and exercise intolerance (defined as $Vo_2max < 25$ mL/kg/min) were randomized to placebo, prazosin, or a combination of isosorbide dinitrate and hydralazine. Vasodilation with this combination showed 36% mortality benefit compared with a control group who received therapy with digoxin and diuretic.[39] Post hoc analysis showed particular benefit among African Americans. These data were later confirmed in the A-HeFT trial, in which more than 1000 African American patients with systolic dysfunction in NYHA class III and IV heart failure, on standard heart failure therapy including β-blockers, ACEI, and ARB, were randomized to placebo or a combination of hydralazine and nitrates.[40] Composite outcomes (death, hospitalization, and quality of life) were better in the treatment group. The beneficial effect of the nitrate/hydralazine combination is believed to be mediated by increased nitric oxide bioavailability. The combination of hydralazine and nitrates is currently reserved for patients who are intolerant of ACEI/ARB and for African Americans who continue to be symptomatic after maximal neurohumoral blockade with β-blockers and ACEI/ARB.

β-BLOCKERS

Long-term inhibition of the sympathetic nervous system with β-blockers has been shown to increase ejection fraction, reduce heart rate, decrease apoptosis, reduce symptoms of heart failure, and also improve overall mortality in patients with both mild and advanced heart failure. β-Blockers also inhibit the renin-angiotensin pathway and further inhibit the neurohumoral pathway. Although many β-blockers are on the market, long-acting metoprolol, carvedilol, and bisoprolol are the only β-blockers that have shown mortality benefit in patients with heart

failure and advanced disease in prospective, randomized, placebo-controlled trials.[41–44] These drugs have been tested in patients with all stages of symptomatic heart failure, showing a mortality benefit in excess of 35% in class IV patients. No head-to-head studies are available to definitively establish the superiority of one β-blocker rather than the other, although some data suggest superiority of carvedilol rather than short-acting metoprolol.[45]

ALDOSTERONE ANTAGONIST

Spironolactone and the selective aldosterone antagonist eplerenone have shown mortality benefit in patients with systolic dysfunction. The RALES (Randomized Aldactone Evaluation Study) trial showed significant mortality benefit in patients with ejection fraction less than 30% and NYHA class III and IV symptoms taking aldactone in addition to ACEIs (**Fig. 3**).[46] In the more recent EMPHASIS-HF (Eplerenone in Mild Patients Hospitalization and Survival Study in Heart Failure) trial, eplerenone improved outcomes in less sick patients with NYHA class II symptoms and ejection fraction less than 35%.[47]

FUNNY CHANNEL INHIBITOR

Ivabradine is an I_f channel inhibitor at the sinoatrial node. When used in patients with moderate to severe heart failure and systolic dysfunction, ivabradine was shown to significantly reduce the combined end point of heart failure readmission and cardiovascular death. This therapy, although

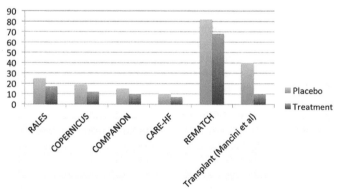

Fig. 3. Twelve-month mortality among placebo and treatment groups for selected trials enrolling patients with advanced heart failure. RALES, The Effect of Spironolactone of Morbidity and Mortality in Patients with Severe Heart Failure[77]; COPERNICUS, The Carvedilol Prospective Randomized Cumulative Survival trial[78]; COMPANION, Cardiac Resynchronization Therapy with or without an Implantable Defibrillator in Advanced Chronic Heart Failure[58]; CARE-HF, The Effect of Cardiac Resynchronization on Morbidity and Mortality in Heart Failure[59]; REMATCH, Long-term Use of a Left Ventricular Assist Device for End-stage Heart Failure[79]; Transplant, value of peak exercise oxygen consumption for optimal timing of cardiac transplantation in ambulatory patients with heart failure.[7]

not currently approved by the US Food and Drug Administration, is available in Europe.[48]

DEVICE THERAPIES
Implantable Cardioverter-Defibrillator Therapy

Risk of sudden cardiac death is high in patients with cardiomyopathy. The risk of cardiovascular mortality is highest in the first 3 months after the initial diagnosis of heart failure, although implantable cardioverter-defibrillator (ICD) therapy has not been shown to be beneficial during this time.[49,50] This may be, in part, because most deaths shortly after initial diagnosis are caused by pump failure rather than arrhythmia. The importance of ICD therapy for secondary prevention of sudden cardiac death is well established based on multiple trials.[51–53] Likewise, the role of ICD therapy in the primary prevention of sudden death has been established among patients with symptomatic heart failure.[54–56] Class IV heart failure was not broadly represented in these studies and the benefit of ICD therapy in this population remains uncertain. However, ICD therapy tested in trials evaluating biventricular pacing has shown benefit in advanced heart failure populations.

Cardiac Resynchronization Therapy

One-third of patients with heart failure have a wide QRS, defined as QRS width greater than 120 milliseconds, which has been associated with poor long-term prognosis. Prolonged QRS duration is often associated with mechanical dyssynchrony, leading to impaired systolic function and altered wall stress. Dyssynchrony is also associated with prolonged and more severe mitral regurgitation and reduced diastolic filling time.[5,57] Resynchronization therapy with placement of an LV/coronary sinus lead has been shown to reduce LV size, improve ejection fraction, and diminish mitral regurgitation jet area. In long-term studies, cardiac resynchronization therapy (CRT) is associated with reduced heart failure hospitalizations and death in patients with NYHA class III and IV heart failure.[58,59]

Recent studies have shown improvement in outcomes in less sick patients with NYHA class 1 to 2 symptoms, which again emphasizes the role of resynchronization therapy in reverse remodeling.[60,61] Patients with left bundle branch block and QRS duration greater than 150 milliseconds have a better chance of responding to resynchronization therapy. Resynchronization therapy is limited by coronary anatomy. Patients with scar tissue, right bundle branch block, mechanical dyssynchrony, and atrial fibrillation have limited benefit from this therapy. Although biventricular pacing has shown clear benefit in stable patients with advanced heart failure, there is no established role for the use of this therapy in patients who seem inotrope dependent.

PREDICTION OF PROGNOSIS

The ability to predict prognosis in heart failure has been widely investigated and is attainable across large groups of patients with matched characteristics. Several prediction models have been developed and validated in large cohorts.[62] However, the values of parameters used to calculate prognosis change with clinical status, making estimation of prognosis a moving target. A willingness to regularly reevaluate prognosis in individual patients at routine intervals is required. Although clinicians may turn to prognostic models in an effort to guide patients' expectations and therapeutic choices at times when the clinical picture worsens, modeling prognosis in unstable patients with heart failure is particularly difficult, and experts agree that clinical prediction tools are less effective in this setting.[63] Despite these challenges, the ability to prognosticate accurately in individuals with advanced heart failure is of critical importance to determine appropriate timing for use of mechanical circulatory support and/or heart transplantation.

Individual Indicators of Adverse Prognosis

A broad array of indices has been correlated with adverse outcome in heart failure (NYHA,[8–10] LVEF,[64] coexisting diastolic dysfunction,[65] RV failure,[66] low peak V_{O_2},[7] low mean arterial pressure,[67] renal dysfunction,[68] and increased diuretic requirements[69]). Many of these factors reflect disarray in the heart failure physiology discussed earlier, whereas others, such as depression,[70] remain poorly understood.

Survival Score

The heart failure survival score (HFSS) was developed to assess stable, ambulatory patients who might be candidates for heart transplant.[5] It is specifically designed to aid in risk assessment for the growing numbers of NYHA class 3 patients who were being listed for heart transplantation during a period of rapid adoption of orthotopic heart transplantation (OHT) as an accepted therapy with excellent outcomes. This score was derived from a cohort of 286 patients evaluated for severe heart failure or for cardiac transplantation. This score was validated in a cohort of 199 patients referred to a different hospital for cardiac transplant evaluation. Ninety individual clinical characteristics known to be associated with adverse outcome in heart failure were evaluated. The most robust predictive model using the fewest variables was sought, leading to the identification of 8 noninvasive and 1 invasive (pulmonary capillary wedge pressure) variable for inclusion in the score. Although the HFSS continues to be used in clinical practice, its value is limited because it was derived before the routine use of β-blockers, aldosterone antagonists, implantable cardiac defibrillators (ICDs), and biventricular pacing treatments. However, unlike the Seattle Heart Failure Model (SHFM), which was derived from patients selected for inclusion in randomized placebo-controlled drug trials, the HFSS was derived from the type of population in which its use was initially imagined: an unselected group of patients referred for assessment for advanced heart failure or for evaluation for cardiac transplantation.

The SHFM

The SHFM was developed to estimate survival in patients with heart failure using readily obtainable data (age, demographics, medications, hemoglobin, lymphocyte percent, uric acid, total cholesterol, and sodium).[6] The model was derived from a cohort of patients enrolled in the Prospective Randomized Amlodipine Survival Evaluation (PRAISE1) study and then validated in 5 separate cohorts derived from other heart failure studies (ELITE2, Val-HeFT, UW, RENAISSANCE, and IN-CHF). A high correlation between predicted and actual survival was shown and varied little between derivation and validation cohorts. The strength of the SHFM model is that it provides reasonable 1-year, 2-year, and 3-year prognostic information and incorporates the effect of all routinely used current heart failure therapies.

Franciosa and Cohn

Early efforts to understand prognosis in advanced heart failure were hampered by lack of systematized prospective approaches. In 1983, before the advent of modern heart failure therapy, widespread mechanical circulatory support, and widespread acceptance of heart transplantation, Franciosa and colleagues,[71] in collaboration with Jay Cohn, authored a seminal paper on survival in men with severe LV failure caused by ischemic disease or idiopathic dilated cardiomyopathy (IDCM). Medical therapy for heart failure during this era was limited to hydralazine and nitrates, digoxin, and diuretics. One-hundred and eighty-two patients were followed prospectively for an average of 12 months. Cases of LV dysfunction from coronary disease were slightly more numerous than LV dysfunction from other causes. Mortality for the group at 1, 2, and 3 years was 34%, 59%, and 76% (**Fig. 4**). Those with coronary disease did significantly worse than those with idiopathic dilated cardiomyopathy (IDCM), although mortality at 2 years was still high (48%) in those with IDCM. Worse heart failure class and hemodynamic abnormalities predicted increased mortality. The investigators then studied whether hemodynamic variables predicting increased mortality also predicted mortality in any given individual. All variables

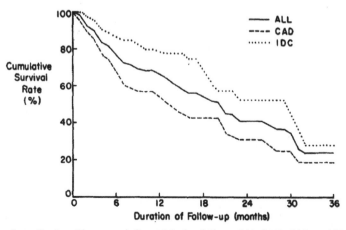

Fig. 4. Survival curves in patients with severe left ventricular failure. ALL, both CAD and IDC groups combined; CAD, coronary artery disease; IDC, idiopathic dilated cardiomyopathy. (*From* Franciosa JA, Wilen M, Ziesche S, et al. Survival in men with severe chronic left ventricular failure due to either coronary heart disease or idiopathic dilated cardiomyopathy. Am J Cardiol 1983;51(5):832; with permission.)

were excluded with the exception of LV end-diastolic pressure, which maintained a weak predictive value. The investigators concluded that mortality was high in patients with severe LV failure, and that those with worse symptoms and hemodynamic abnormalities fared poorly, but cautioned that individual hemodynamic variables are of limited value in the prognosis of individual patients.

Evidence for Improved Prognosis in Heart Failure Since Franciosa and Cohn

Analysis of large data sets from the Framingham Study, the Mayo Clinic, and Medicare have shown improvement in prognosis among patients with heart failure with time (**Table 2**).[72–74] The degree of improvement has been less obvious in specialized populations, particularly among the elderly.[75,76] These trends may reflect improvements in heart failure therapy, although the magnitude of benefit is less robust than might be expected given the results of randomized studies evaluating specific therapies. As opposed to populations selected for inclusion in randomized controlled studies, patients represented in the data sets mentioned earlier are more heterogeneous and likely to suffer more severely from a wider array of comorbidities, which leads to a watering-down effect that diminishes the measurable benefit of heart failure therapies but also to a more realistic assessment of gains made by medical heart failure therapy.

Franciosa and Cohn versus Population-based Outcome Studies

Outcomes among the patients in Franciosa's work were markedly worse than those in the population-based studies noted earlier, which likely reflects differences in the severity of heart failure among participants. The Framingham and Mayo populations were selected without regard to severity of heart failure, and without regard to cause. Included in these cohorts are patients with mild heart failure, and those with primarily diastolic heart failure. The Scottish study included a sicker group of patients, because they were identified by incident hospitalization. However, this study was not structured to specify the cause or severity of heart failure.

Survival Data from Patients with Advanced Heart Failure

As reviewed earlier, randomized controlled trials assessing the value of both medical and electrophysiologic (ICD and CRT) therapies have shown consistent reduction in mortality among control and treatment groups as therapies have been stacked (see **Fig. 3**). Application of the SHFM to patients with advanced heart failure similarly predicts improved outcome with the use of medical and electrophysiologic therapies. These data are supported by analysis of changes in prognosis among patients listed for heart transplantation between the 1990 to 1994 and 2000 to 2005 eras. In an elegant study, data from the OPTN/UNOS database was analyzed for changes in prognosis, and risk factors associated with poor prognosis, among patients listed for heart transplantation, broken down by listing status (1, most precarious, vs 2, less precarious). One-year survival improved from 49.5% to 60% among the sickest patients (status 1), and 81.8% to 89.4% among stable outpatients (status 2). Franciosa and Cohn's population may be comparable with patients listed as status 2 for heart transplantation, because these patients are typified by systolic heart failure with refractory symptoms not requiring continuous inotrope infusion. Although this comparison is imperfect, doubling of 1-year survival in the early cohort with continued improvement in the subsequent decade may be interpreted as reflecting the effect of medical, and later electrophysiologic, therapies in patients with advanced heart failure caused by LV systolic failure.

SUMMARY

Despite improvements in prognosis since Franciosa and Cohn's publication, advanced heart failure caused by systolic failure of the left ventricle remains associated with high mortality. Early and aggressive attempts at establishing a compensated clinical status with institution of medical and appropriate electrophysiologic therapies are the requisite first steps in caring for individuals with advanced heart failure. At the same time, recognition of the high mortality associated with advanced heart failure should prompt physicians to proceed with early assessment for possible use of mechanical cardiac support and

Table 2
Trends in 5-year mortality after diagnosis of heart failure

Study	Number of Patients	Before 1990 (%)	After 1990 (%)
Framingham	1075	Female 57 Male 70	Female 45 Male 59
Mayo Clinic	4537	Female 51 Male 65	Female 46 Male 50

heart transplantation, so that timely application of these therapies is possible when medical therapy fails.

REFERENCES

1. Writing Group Members, Lloyd-Jones D, Adams RJ, et al. Heart disease and stroke statistics–2010 update: a report from the American Heart Association. Circulation 2010;121(7):e46–215.

2. Writing Committee Members, Hunt SA, Abraham WT, et al. 2009 focused update incorporated into the ACC/AHA 2005 guidelines for the diagnosis and management of heart failure in adults: a report of the American College of Cardiology Foundation/American Heart Association Task Force on practice guidelines: developed in collaboration with the International Society for Heart and Lung Transplantation. Circulation 2009;119(14):e391–479.

3. Okura Y, Urban LH, Mahoney DW, et al. Agreement between self-report questionnaires and medical record data was substantial for diabetes, hypertension, myocardial infarction and stroke but not for heart failure. J Clin Epidemiol 2004;57(10):1096–103.

4. Mehra MR, Kobashigawa J, Starling R, et al. Listing criteria for heart transplantation: International Society for Heart and Lung Transplantation guidelines for the care of cardiac transplant candidates–2006. J Heart Lung Transplant 2006;25(9):1024–42.

5. Aaronson KD, Schwartz JS, Chen TM, et al. Development and prospective validation of a clinical index to predict survival in ambulatory patients referred for cardiac transplant evaluation. Circulation 1997;95(12):2660–7.

6. Levy WC, Mozaffarian D, Linker DT, et al. The Seattle Heart Failure Model: prediction of survival in heart failure. Circulation 2006;113(11):1424–33.

7. Mancini DM, Eisen H, Kussmaul W, et al. Value of peak exercise oxygen consumption for optimal timing of cardiac transplantation in ambulatory patients with heart failure. Circulation 1991;83(3):778–86.

8. Effect of enalapril on mortality and the development of heart failure in asymptomatic patients with reduced left ventricular ejection fractions. The SOLVD Investigators. N Engl J Med 1992;327(10):685–91.

9. Effect of enalapril on survival in patients with reduced left ventricular ejection fractions and congestive heart failure. The SOLVD Investigators. N Engl J Med 1991;325(5):293–302.

10. Effects of enalapril on mortality in severe congestive heart failure. Results of the Cooperative North Scandinavian Enalapril Survival Study (CONSENSUS). The CONSENSUS Trial Study Group. N Engl J Med 1987;316(23):1429–35.

11. Mann DL, Bristow MR. Mechanisms and models in heart failure: the biomechanical model and beyond (vol 111, pg 2837, 2005). Circulation 2005;112(4):E75.

12. Eisenhofer G, Friberg P, Rundqvist B, et al. Cardiac sympathetic nerve function in congestive heart failure. Circulation 1996;93(9):1667–76.

13. Kameda K, Matsunaga T, Abe N, et al. Correlation of oxidative stress with activity of matrix metalloproteinase in patients with coronary artery disease. Possible role for left ventricular remodelling. Eur Heart J 2003;24(24):2180–5.

14. Beuckelmann DJ, Nabauer M, Erdmann E. Intracellular calcium handling in isolated ventricular myocytes from patients with terminal heart failure. Circulation 1992;85(3):1046–55.

15. Olivetti G, Abbi R, Quaini F, et al. Apoptosis in the failing human heart. N Engl J Med 1997;336(16):1131–41.

16. Weber KT, Brilla CG, Janicki JS. Myocardial fibrosis: functional significance and regulatory factors. Cardiovasc Res 1993;27(3):341–8.

17. Mann DL, Bristow MR. Mechanisms and models in heart failure: the biomechanical model and beyond. Circulation 2005;111(21):2837–49.

18. Mettauer B, Zoll J, Garnier A, et al. Heart failure: a model of cardiac and skeletal muscle energetic failure. Pflugers Arch 2006;452(6):653–66.

19. Mancini DM, Walter G, Reichek N, et al. Contribution of skeletal muscle atrophy to exercise intolerance and altered muscle metabolism in heart failure. Circulation 1992;85(4):1364–73.

20. Jiang W, Kuchibhatla M, Clary GL, et al. Relationship between depressive symptoms and long-term mortality in patients with heart failure. Am Heart J 2007;154(1):102–8.

21. Dunbar SB, Heo S, Pressler SJ, et al. Abstract 2092: heart failure patients with diabetes have more co-morbidities and self care problems. Circulation 2008;118(18_Meeting Abstracts):S_668.

22. Lahiri MK, Kannankeril PJ, Goldberger JJ. Assessment of autonomic function in cardiovascular disease: physiological basis and prognostic implications. J Am Coll Cardiol 2008;51(18):1725–33.

23. Triposkiadis F, Karayannis G, Giamouzis G, et al. The sympathetic nervous system in heart failure: physiology, pathophysiology, and clinical implications. J Am Coll Cardiol 2009;54(19):1747–62.

24. Weber KT. Aldosterone in congestive heart failure. N Engl J Med 2001;345(23):1689–97.

25. Kostin S, Pool L, Elsasser A, et al. Myocytes die by multiple mechanisms in failing human hearts. Circ Res 2003;92(7):715–24.

26. Keith M, Geranmayegan A, Sole M, et al. Increased oxidative stress in patients with congestive heart failure. J Am Coll Cardiol 1998;31(6):1352–6.

27. Giordano FJ. Oxygen, oxidative stress, hypoxia, and heart failure. J Clin Invest 2005;115(3):500–8.

28. Cheng W, Li B, Kajstura J, et al. Stretch-induced programmed myocyte cell death. J Clin Invest 1995;96(5):2247–59.

29. Anker SD, Chua TP, Ponikowski P, et al. Hormonal changes and catabolic/anabolic imbalance in chronic heart failure and their importance for cardiac cachexia. Circulation 1997;96(2):526–34.

30. Guiha NH, Cohn JN, Mikulic E, et al. Treatment of refractory heart failure with infusion of nitroprusside. N Engl J Med 1974;291(12):587–92.

31. Cohn JN, Franciosa JA. Vasodilator therapy of cardiac failure (second of two parts). N Engl J Med 1977;297(5):254–8.

32. Pierpont GL, Cohn JN, Franciosa JA. Combined oral hydralazine-nitrate therapy in left ventricular failure. Hemodynamic equivalency to sodium nitroprusside. Chest 1978;73(1):8–13.

33. Cohn JN, Levine TB, Francis GS, et al. Neurohumoral control mechanisms in congestive heart failure. Am Heart J 1981;102(3 Pt 2):509–14.

34. Grassi G, Cattaneo BM, Seravalle G, et al. Effects of chronic ACE inhibition on sympathetic nerve traffic and baroreflex control of circulation in heart failure. Circulation 1997;96(4):1173–9.

35. Gibbs CR, Blann AD, Watson RD, et al. Abnormalities of hemorheological, endothelial, and platelet function in patients with chronic heart failure in sinus rhythm-effects of angiotensin-converting enzyme inhibitor and beta-blocker therapy. Circulation 2001;103(13):1746–51.

36. Vaughan DE, Rouleau JL, Ridker PM, et al. Effects of ramipril on plasma fibrinolytic balance in patients with acute anterior myocardial infarction. Circulation 1997;96(2):442–7.

37. Cohn JN, Tognoni G. A randomized trial of the angiotensin-receptor blocker valsartan in chronic heart failure. N Engl J Med 2001;345(23):1667–75.

38. Granger CB, McMurray JJ, Yusuf S, et al. Effects of candesartan in patients with chronic heart failure and reduced left-ventricular systolic function intolerant to angiotensin-converting-enzyme inhibitors: the CHARM-Alternative trial. Lancet 2003;362(9386):772–6.

39. Cohn JN, Archibald DG, Ziesche S, et al. Effect of vasodilator therapy on mortality in chronic congestive heart failure. Results of a Veterans Administration Cooperative study. N Engl J Med 1986;314(24):1547–52.

40. Taylor AL, Ziesche S, Yancy C, et al. Combination of isosorbide dinitrate and hydralazine in blacks with heart failure. N Engl J Med 2004;351(20):2049–57.

41. Effect of metoprolol CR/XL in chronic heart failure: Metoprolol CR/XL Randomised Intervention Trial in Congestive Heart Failure (MERIT-HF). Lancet 1999;353(9169):2001–7.

42. The Cardiac Insufficiency Bisoprolol Study II (CIBIS-II): a randomised trial. Lancet 1999;353(9146):9–13.

43. Packer M, Bristow MR, Cohn JN, et al. The effect of carvedilol on morbidity and mortality in patients with chronic heart failure. U.S. Carvedilol Heart Failure Study Group. N Engl J Med 1996;334(21):1349–55.

44. Waagstein F, Bristow MR, Swedberg K, et al. Beneficial effects of metoprolol in idiopathic dilated cardiomyopathy. Metoprolol in Dilated Cardiomyopathy (MDC) Trial Study Group. Lancet 1993;342(8885):1441–6.

45. Poole-Wilson PA, Swedberg K, Cleland JG, et al. Comparison of carvedilol and metoprolol on clinical outcomes in patients with chronic heart failure in the Carvedilol or Metoprolol European Trial (COMET): randomised controlled trial. Lancet 2003;362(9377):7–13.

46. Schwinger RH. The aldosterone antagonist spironolactone prolongs the survival of chronic heart failure patients. The results of the RALES study. The Randomized Aldactone Evaluation Study. Dtsch Med Wochenschr 1999;124(34–35):987–8 [in German].

47. Zannad F, McMurray JJ, Krum H, et al. Eplerenone in patients with systolic heart failure and mild symptoms. N Engl J Med 2011;364(1):11–21.

48. Swedberg K, Komajda M, Bohm M, et al. Ivabradine and outcomes in chronic heart failure (SHIFT): a randomised placebo-controlled study. Lancet 2010;376(9744):875–85.

49. Hohnloser SH, Kuck KH, Dorian P, et al. Prophylactic use of an implantable cardioverter-defibrillator after acute myocardial infarction. N Engl J Med 2004;351(24):2481–8.

50. Bigger JT Jr. Prophylactic use of implanted cardiac defibrillators in patients at high risk for ventricular arrhythmias after coronary-artery bypass graft surgery. Coronary Artery Bypass Graft (CABG) Patch Trial Investigators. N Engl J Med 1997;337(22):1569–75.

51. A comparison of antiarrhythmic-drug therapy with implantable defibrillators in patients resuscitated from near-fatal ventricular arrhythmias. The Antiarrhythmics versus Implantable Defibrillators (AVID) Investigators. N Engl J Med 1997;337(22):1576–83.

52. Kuck KH, Cappato R, Siebels J, et al. Randomized comparison of antiarrhythmic drug therapy with implantable defibrillators in patients resuscitated from cardiac arrest: the Cardiac Arrest Study Hamburg (CASH). Circulation 2000;102(7):748–54.

53. Connolly SJ, Gent M, Roberts RS, et al. Canadian implantable defibrillator study (CIDS): a randomized trial of the implantable cardioverter defibrillator against amiodarone. Circulation 2000;101(11):1297–302.

54. Moss AJ, Hall WJ, Cannom DS, et al. Improved survival with an implanted defibrillator in patients with coronary disease at high risk for ventricular arrhythmia. Multicenter Automatic Defibrillator

Implantation Trial Investigators. N Engl J Med 1996; 335(26):1933–40.

55. Moss AJ, Zareba W, Hall WJ, et al. Prophylactic implantation of a defibrillator in patients with myocardial infarction and reduced ejection fraction. N Engl J Med 2002;346(12):877–83.

56. Bardy GH, Lee KL, Mark DB, et al. Amiodarone or an implantable cardioverter-defibrillator for congestive heart failure. N Engl J Med 2005;352(3):225–37.

57. Grines CL, Bashore TM, Boudoulas H, et al. Functional abnormalities in isolated left bundle branch block. The effect of interventricular asynchrony. Circulation 1989;79(4):845–53.

58. Bristow MR, Saxon LA, Boehmer J, et al. Cardiac-resynchronization therapy with or without an implantable defibrillator in advanced chronic heart failure. N Engl J Med 2004;350(21):2140–50.

59. Cleland JG, Daubert JC, Erdmann E, et al. The effect of cardiac resynchronization on morbidity and mortality in heart failure. N Engl J Med 2005;352(15): 1539–49.

60. Moss AJ, Hall WJ, Cannom DS, et al. Cardiac-resynchronization therapy for the prevention of heart-failure events. N Engl J Med 2009;361(14):1329–38.

61. Linde C, Abraham WT, Gold MR, et al. Randomized trial of cardiac resynchronization in mildly symptomatic heart failure patients and in asymptomatic patients with left ventricular dysfunction and previous heart failure symptoms. J Am Coll Cardiol 2008; 52(23):1834–43.

62. Adler ED, Goldfinger JZ, Kalman J, et al. Palliative care in the treatment of advanced heart failure. Circulation 2009;120(25):2597–606.

63. Goldberg LR, Jessup M. A time to be born and a time to die. Circulation 2007;116(4):360–2.

64. Wong M, Staszewsky L, Latini R, et al. Severity of left ventricular remodeling defines outcomes and response to therapy in heart failure: Valsartan Heart Failure Trial (Val-HeFT) echocardiographic data. J Am Coll Cardiol 2004;43(11):2022–7.

65. Pinamonti B, Di Lenarda A, Sinagra G, et al. Restrictive left ventricular filling pattern in dilated cardiomyopathy assessed by Doppler echocardiography: clinical, echocardiographic and hemodynamic correlations and prognostic implications. Heart Muscle Disease Study Group. J Am Coll Cardiol 1993;22(3): 808–15.

66. Ghio S, Gavazzi A, Campana C, et al. Independent and additive prognostic value of right ventricular systolic function and pulmonary artery pressure in patients with chronic heart failure. J Am Coll Cardiol 2001;37(1):183–8.

67. Domanski MJ, Mitchell GF, Norman J, et al. Independent prognostic information provided by sphygmomanometrically determined pulse pressure and mean arterial pressure in patients with left ventricular dysfunction. Circulation 1998;98(17):225.

68. Dries DL, Exner DV, Domanski MJ, et al. The prognostic implications of renal insufficiency in asymptomatic and symptomatic patients with left ventricular systolic dysfunction. J Am Coll Cardiol 2000;35(3): 681–9.

69. Neuberg GW, Miller AB, O'Connor CM, et al. Diuretic resistance predicts mortality in patients with advanced heart failure. Am Heart J 2002;144(1): 31–8.

70. Jiang W, Kuchibhatla M, Cuffe MS, et al. Prognostic value of anxiety and depression in patients with chronic heart failure. Circulation 2004;110(22): 3452–6.

71. Franciosa JA, Wilen M, Ziesche S, et al. Survival in men with severe chronic left ventricular failure due to either coronary heart disease or idiopathic dilated cardiomyopathy. Am J Cardiol 1983;51(5):831–6.

72. Baker DW, Einstadter D, Thomas C, et al. Mortality trends for 23,505 Medicare patients hospitalized with heart failure in Northeast Ohio, 1991 to 1997. Am Heart J 2003;146(2):258–64.

73. Levy D, Kenchaiah S, Larson MG, et al. Long-term trends in the incidence of and survival with heart failure. N Engl J Med 2002;347(18):1397–402.

74. Roger VL, Weston SA, Redfield MM, et al. Trends in heart failure incidence and survival in a community-based population. JAMA 2004;292(3):344–50.

75. Curtis LH, Greiner MA, Hammill BG, et al. Early and long-term outcomes of heart failure in elderly persons, 2001-2005. Arch Intern Med 2008;168(22): 2481–8.

76. Kosiborod M, Lichtman JH, Heidenreich PA, et al. National trends in outcomes among elderly patients with heart failure. Am J Med 2006;119(7):616.e1–7.

77. Pitt B, Zannad F, Remme WJ, et al. The effect of spironolactone on morbidity and mortality in patients with severe heart failure. Randomized Aldactone Evaluation Study Investigators. N Engl J Med 1999;341(10):709–17.

78. Eichhorn EJ, Bristow MR. The Carvedilol Prospective Randomized Cumulative Survival (COPERNICUS) trial. Curr Control Trials Cardiovasc Med 2001;2(1): 20–3.

79. Rose EA, Gelijns AC, Moskowitz AJ, et al. Long-term use of a left ventricular assist device for end-stage heart failure. N Engl J Med 2001;345(20): 1435–43.

Editorial Comment on "Natural History of End-Stage LV Dysfunction: Has it Improved from the Classic Franciosa and Cohn Graph?"

John A. Elefteriades, MD

KEY MESSAGES

In "Natural History of End-Stage LV Dysfunction: Has It Improved from the Classic Franciosa and Cohn Graph?" Dr Daniel Jacoby and colleagues argue that prognosis of patients with heart failure has indeed improved since the landmark dismal depiction nearly 3 decades ago in the classic graph by Franciosa and Cohn (76% mortality at 3 years). Dr Jacoby and colleagues attribute this improvement in outlook to the advent of effective heart failure therapies, including angiotensin-converting enzyme inhibitors, β-blockers, aldosterone inhibitors, cardiac resynchronization therapy, and the implantable cardioverter defibrillator.

STRENGTHS

The investigators point effectively to large-scale clinical trials that have demonstrated convincingly the effectiveness of the therapies listed.

WEAKNESSES

As the investigators point out, in real-life populations from Framingham, Mayo, and Medicare databases, "these trends reflect improvements in heart failure therapy, though the magnitude of benefit is less robust than might be expected [from] randomized studies evaluating specific therapies."[1] The mortality for medical management of advanced heart failure (ischemic or idiopathic) remains high, mandating aggressive application of mechanical cardiac augmentation therapies and heart transplantation.

REFERENCE

1. Jacoby D, Albajrami O, Bellumkonda L. Natural history of end-stage LV dysfunction: has it improved from the classic Franciosa and Cohn graph? Cardiol Clin, in press.

Section of Cardiac Surgery, Yale University School of Medicine, Boardman 2, 333 Cedar Street, New Haven, CT 06510, USA
E-mail address: john.elefteriades@yale.edu

Cardiol Clin 29 (2011) 497
doi:10.1016/j.ccl.2011.08.009
0733-8651/11/$ – see front matter © 2011 Elsevier Inc. All rights reserved.

Current Technology: Devices Available for Destination Therapy

Hiroo Takayama, MD, Jonathan A. Yang, MD,
Yoshifumi Naka, MD, PhD*

KEYWORDS

- Destination therapy • HeartMate XVE • HeartMate II
- HeartWare

A new era of end-stage heart failure (HF) treatment with left ventricular assist device (LVAD) technology has emerged with 2 landmark randomized control trials. The first trial, the Randomized Evaluation of Mechanical Assistance for the Treatment of Congestive Heart Failure (REMATCH) trial, validated the feasibility of a mechanical approach to the treatment of end-stage HF in 2001.[1] This trial led to the first approval by the US Food and Drug Administration (FDA) of an LVAD therapy for destination therapy (DT) with the HeartMate (HM) XVE. The second trial was completed recently and reported that the probability of survival free from stroke and device failure at 2 years was significantly improved on a continuous flow (CF) pump (HM II) compared with a pulsatile flow (PF) pump (HM XVE) in DT patients.[2] The FDA approved this CF LVAD for DT in 2010. The HM XVE and the HM II are the only 2 FDA-approved devices currently and have set the standards for LVAD use as DT. Several other devices are or will soon be undergoing clinical trials in the United States.

PF LVADs

LVADs are divided into PF and CF devices based on the characteristics of blood flow generated by the pump. The first-generation LVADs are characterized by a volume displacement pump that generates PF. In addition to the REMATCH trial, the Investigation of Nontransplant-Eligible Patients Who Are Inotrope Dependent (INTrEPID) trial and the European LionHeart Clinical Utility Baseline Study (CUBS) trial evaluated the use of the Novacor LVAD and the Arrow LionHeart LVAD, respectively.[3,4] All of these clinical trials revealed superior outcomes of PF LVADs over medical therapy for end-stage HF. However, widespread use of these LVADs for DT did not occur because of limitations highlighted by their high incidence of adverse events related to mechanical support, such as infection, device failure, and thromboembolic events, as well as their bulky and noisy design.

The HM XVE (Thoratec Corp. Pleasanton, CA, USA) (Fig. 1) was developed by Thermo Cardiosystems and is currently manufactured by Thoratec Corp. The original pump was operated with a pneumatic power source (the IP model). This model evolved into the vented electric (VE) model and then to the XVE model. The XVE model has improved strength of the percutaneous lead and an outflow graft with bend relief; also, the mounting of its biologic valve prosthesis is enhanced, as well as some other refinements. This device generates PF through a pusher plate situated in a relatively large housing, which precludes implantation in small patients (body surface area <1.5 kg/m^2). The unique textured inner surface of the titanium shell with a polyurethane diaphragm decreases the thrombogenic nature of the device, allowing patient

Yoshifumi Naka receives consultant fee from Thoratec and DuraHeart. The other authors have nothing to disclose.
Department of Surgery, Columbia University Medical Center, Milstein Hospital Building, 7-435, 177 Fort Washington Avenue, New York, NY 10032, USA
* Corresponding author.
E-mail address: yn33@columbia.edu

Cardiol Clin 29 (2011) 499–504
doi:10.1016/j.ccl.2011.08.005
0733-8651/11/$ – see front matter © 2011 Published by Elsevier Inc.

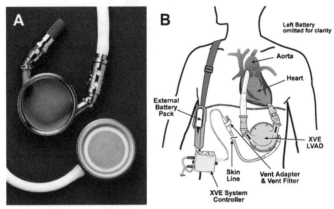

Fig. 1. (*A*) The pump of the HM XVE. The unique textured inner surface of the titanium shell with a polyurethane diaphragm decreases the thrombogenic nature of the device (*B*). (*Courtesy of* Thoratec Corp.)

management with no anticoagulation. A pusher-plate actuator produces mechanical energy converted from electrical energy. The inflow and outflow arms extend from the pump, and each arm contains a 25-mm porcine valve. The inflow cannula is placed into the left ventricular (LV) cavity through a plastic cuff sewn at the LV apex. The outflow arm is connected to a 20-mm Dacron graft, which is sewn to the ascending aorta in end-to-side fashion. The pump is placed in a large pocket in the anterior abdomen (in either the preperitoneal or the intraperitoneal space) and the percutaneous lead is brought out in the lower abdominal wall. Although the VE and the XVE models operate on electric energy, the percutaneous driveline contains a duct that allows access to the diaphragm and can be used for venting or pneumatic actuation of the device in emergent situations such as electrical driver failure. The driveline is connected to an external controller that weighs less than 300 g and to 2 batteries.

This device successfully pioneered a new era in HF therapy. The REMATCH trial randomly compared the HM VE with optimal medical management for patients with end-stage HF who were ineligible for heart transplantation (HTx).[1] It showed that survival at 1 and 2 years was 52% and 23% with the LVAD compared with 25% and 8%, respectively, with medical therapy. However, long-term use is limited by significant rate of device malfunction and infection. In the REMATCH study, the probability of device-related infection was reported to be 28% within 3 months, and that of device failure was 35% at 24 months. Although subsequent clinical studies have shown a better safety profile and greater reliability of the updated device (XVE), the average support that the pump can offer remains around 1.5 years.[5] Lietz and colleagues[6] reported the outcomes of this device in the post-REMATCH era. That study

included 280 patients who underwent HM XVE LVAD implantation between November 2001 and December 2005 and reported that the probability of device exchange or fatal device failure was 72.9% at 2 years. Given these limitations and the recent approval of the HM II (Thoratec Corp, Pleasanton, CA, USA) for DT, the role for the HM XVE in DT is now minimal. A potential continued indication for its use remains in patients who have contraindications for anticoagulation; however, durability remains a major concern.

Another widely used PF device was the Novacor LVAS. Its basic mechanism is similar to that of the HM XVE but with a smoother inner surface, which anecdotally requires stringent anticoagulation. This device, although used worldwide for bridge to transplant (BTT), had a slightly higher incidence of stroke, This device was a durable workhorse for many years, and the stroke issue was improved with a new inflow cannula.[7] Nonetheless, sale of the Novacor was discontinued in 2008. No clinical trial using a PF device for DT is currently ongoing or being planned.

CF LVADs

Second-generation LVADs are characterized by CF driven by a rotary pump. This technology has proved more mechanically reliable and better tolerated by patients. In particular, the HM II (**Fig. 2**), was shown in a randomized control trial to be superior to the HM XVE for DT patients.[2] This device was the second to receive FDA approval for DT in January 2010, which led to rapid expansion of its clinical application. The Interagency Registry for Mechanically Assisted Circulatory Support (INTERMACS) LVAD registry reported 176 HM II implantations for DT during the first 6 months of 2010, a significant increase from 17 during the previous 6 months.[8]

A

B

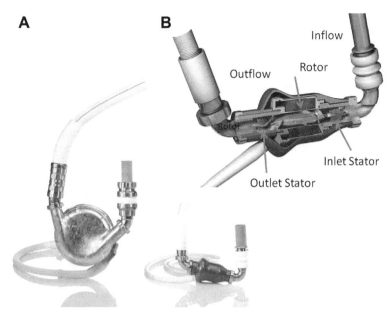

Inflow

Outflow   Rotor

Rotor

Inlet Stator

Outlet Stator

Fig. 2. (*A*) The size difference of the pump for the HM XVE (*left*) and the HM II (*right*). (*B*) The structure of the HM II pump. The rotor is supported by a stator at each end. The only bearings in the device are the 2 for these 2 stators. The electric energy from the driveline is converted to magnetic energy, which then rotates the rotor. The blood is propelled with the centrifugal force created by the rotor and is redirected into axial flow by the stator at the outlet. (*Courtesy of* Thoratec Corp.)

The CF of the HM II is driven by a small axial pump, which weighs 350 g, is 7 cm long, and 4 cm in diameter. The percutaneous driveline is significantly smaller than that of the HM XVE. The rotor rotates at 6000 to 15,000 rpm, generating up to 10 L/min of flow. The rotor, which is contained in titanium housing, is supported by a stator at each end. The only bearings in the device are for these 2 stators. The electrical energy from the driveline is converted to magnetic energy, which then rotates the rotor. The blood is propelled with the centrifugal force created by the rotor and is redirected into axial flow by the stator at the outlet. The 14-mm outflow graft is sewn to the ascending aorta in end-to-side fashion. These design changes allowed for significant miniaturization of mechanical support technology, limiting the surface area exposed to blood, and allowed for the elimination of valves, air vents, and compliance chambers. The presence of fewer moving parts reduces device malfunction rates. Inflow and outflow arms are attached to this pump. The cuff, through which the inflow cannula is inserted into the LV, is the same cuff as the one for the HM XVE to facilitate device exchange. The joint in the inflow arm allows appropriate positioning of the inflow cannula into the LV at the time of implantation as well as synchronous movement with the heartbeat after implantation.

Results from the randomized controlled trial that showed HM II superiority over HM XVE in end-stage HF patients who were ineligible for HTx were recently released by the HM II Investigators.[2] Patients were randomly assigned to an HM II or an HM XVE in a 2:1 ratio, enrolling 134 and 66 patients, respectively. The HM II achieved superior actuarial survival rates at 2 years (58% vs 24%). Pump replacement was necessary in only 9% of the HM II group compared with 34% of the HM XVE group. The leading causes of death among patients receiving an HM II were hemorrhagic stroke (in 9% who underwent device implantation), right HF (in 5%), sepsis (in 4%), external power interruption (in 4%), respiratory failure (in 3%), cardiac arrest (in 3%), and bleeding (in 3%). Among patients receiving an HM XVE, the leading causes of death were hemorrhagic stroke (in 10% who underwent device implantation), right-sided HF (in 8%), multisystem organ failure (in 7%), and ischemic stroke (in 5%). Major adverse events among patients receiving an HM II were significantly lower, including device-related infection (relating to the percutaneous lead, pump, or pump pocket), non–device-related infection, right-sided HF, respiratory failure, renal failure, and cardiac arrhythmia. There was a 38% relative reduction in the rate of rehospitalization in the HM II group compared with those in the HM XVE group. The incidence of stroke did not differ significantly between the HM II and the HM XVE patients (17% vs 14%). The broader and long-term outcomes with real-world use of the HM II remain to be seen. However, the recent third annual report from the INTERMACS registry looked into the survival after LVAD implantation for DT and reported improved 1-year survival of 74% with CF LVADs compared with 61% with PF LVADs, although the follow-up remains short.[8]

Exposure of patients to nonphysiologic CF might cause deleterious effects on end-organ function, and this is of particular concern for patients receiving an LVAD as DT. A recent study compared renal and hepatic function at up to 3 months in 3 groups of patients who were supported by a centrifugal flow LVAD (VentrAssist, n = 10), an axial flow LVAD (HM II, n = 30), or a PF LVAD (HM XVE, n = 18).[9] Among the 3 groups, age, gender, weight, duration of LVAD support, and cause of HF were comparable. No significant differences were found between groups with respect to baseline renal function, hepatic function, or hematologic function. At 1 and 3 months of follow-up, renal and hepatic function either improved or remained within normal limits in all groups. The speed of the HM II was limited to maintain the aortic valve-opening every third beat, and this maintained some pulsatility in the CF LVAD patients, who had a mean pulse pressure range of 27.0 ± 12 to 31.7 ± 17.7, although this was significantly less than that of the PF LVAD patients, which ranged from 55.8 ± 18.8 to 56.9 ± 14.8. Russell and colleagues[10] evaluated renal and hepatic function in 309 patients who had been supported with the HM II for BTT. The patients were divided into those with above-normal and normal laboratory values before implantation, and blood chemistry was measured during HM II support. There were significant improvements over 6 months in all parameters in the above-normal groups, with values in the normal groups remaining in the normal range over time. Mean blood urea nitrogen and serum creatinine in the above-normal groups decreased significantly from 37 ± 14 to 23 ± 10 mg/dL (P<.0001) and from 1.8 ± 0.4 to 1.4 ± 0.8 mg/dL (P<.01), respectively. There were decreases in aspartate transaminase and alanine transaminase in the above-normal groups from 121 ± 206 and 171 ± 348 to 36 ± 19 and 31 ± 22 IU (P<.001), respectively. Total bilirubin for the above-normal group was 2.1 ± 0.9 mg/dL at baseline; after an acute increase at week 1, it decreased to 0.9 ± 0.5 mg/dL by 6 months (P<.0001). These values from patients in the normal groups remained normal during HM II support.

Neurocognitive changes with HM II support were studied by the HM II Investigators by using a neurocognitive protocol to evaluate patient performance (visual spatial perception, auditory and visual memory, executive functions, language and processing speed) at 1, 3, and 6 months after HM II implantation.[11] A total of 239 test sessions were completed in 93 patients. They showed statistically significant improvements between 1, 3, and 6 months in neurocognitive domain performance. Initial concerns over the potential influence of the CF feature on patient physiology seem to have been assuaged based on these midterm outcomes. Although the concerns are based on previous research showing that PF is superior to non-PF, arterial pulsatility is present with CF LVAD support under most clinical conditions, and CF LVADs are not nonpulsatile devices in this sense.

Although the HM II has been repeatedly shown to be superior to the HM XVE, it remains far from ideal for DT application, which requires higher expectations compared with that required for BTT devices. DT devices are exposed to prolonged durations of support and are to have minimum interference with the patient's quality of life. As described earlier, studies still show a significant incidence of device-related infection.[2] The risk of stroke does not seem to be reduced compared with the HM XVE.[2] In addition to these well-recognized issues, we have reported some previously unknown complications related to this technology. The first is the development of aortic insufficiency (AI). We examined preoperative and postoperative echocardiograms of 67 HM I (VE or XVE) and 63 HM II patients who received implants without an aortic valve procedure between January 2004 and September 2009.[12] AI of at least mild severity developed in 4 of the 67 HM I (6.0%) and in 9 of the 63 HM II patients (14.3%). The median times to AI development were 48 days for HM I patients and 90 days for HM II patients. For patients who remained on device support at 6 and 12 months, freedom from AI was 94.5% and 88.9% in HM I patients and 83.6% and 75.2% in HM II patients. Aortic root circumference was assessed in the explant specimen of 77 patients who underwent HTx after LVAD bridge and were significantly larger in HM II patients who had developed AI compared with those who did not (8.44 ± 0.89 vs 7.36 ± 1.02 cm; P = .034). AI was more common in patients whose aortic valve did not open (11 of 26 vs 1 of 14; P = .03). The same concern was raised from a different institution as well. Cowger and colleagues[13] reviewed echocardiograms (n = 315) from 78 patients undergoing HM XVE (n = 25 [32%]) or HM II (n = 53 [68%]) implantation from 2004 to 2008. At 6 months, 89 ± 4% of subjects (n = 49 at risk) were free from moderate or worse AI, but this was reduced to 74 ± 7% (n = 29 at risk) and

49 ± 13% (n = 13 at risk) by 12 and 18 months, respectively. The use of an HM II device was associated with this AI progression.

Another significant complication related to HM II is bleeding. Of 79 patients who received an HM II at our program, 44.3% had bleeding events at 112 ± 183 days after implantation.[14,15] Gastrointestinal bleeding was the most frequent event. Anticoagulation was achieved with warfarin in 68.3%, aspirin in 55.7%, and dipyridamole in 58.2% of the patients. Furthermore, high molecular weight von Willebrand factor multimers were measured in 31 HM II patients and were reduced in all patients, suggesting development of acquired von Willebrand disease in these patients. These complications are unlikely to be specific to HM II but rather related to CF technology.

Another device currently undergoing a clinical trial for DT use is HeartWare LVAD (**Fig. 3**). The detailed description of this device is beyond the scope of this article, but the main feature of the HeartWare LVAD (HeartWare, Inc, Framingham, MA, USA) is its small pump, which allows intrapericardial implantation. The impeller of the pump is a centrifugal pump, suspended within the housing without any mechanical contact by magnets and a hydrodynamic thrust bearing. It can generate up to 10 L/min of flow. The result of a pivotal trial testing its feasibility for BTT use was reported at the American Heart Association 2010. At 180 days after the implantation, 92.0% of the patients with the HeartWare LVAD (n = 137) achieved the primary end point (survival, successful HTx, or device explantation as a result of myocardial recovery). Survival of the patients at 360 days was 90.6% with improvement of the quality of life and 6-minute walk test. Nonrandomized comparison with the HM II group (n = 499) showed noninferiority. These results were received by HF care providers with enthusiasm, and the device is undergoing a trial for DT use.

Although it is not the focus of this article, the improvement in preoperative and postoperative patient care is as important as, if not more important than, the differences and advances in the

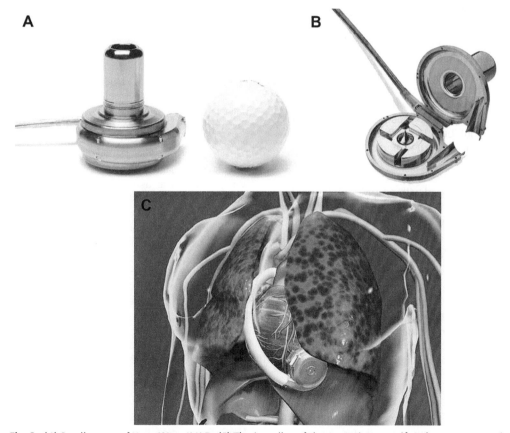

Fig. 3. (*A*) Small pump of HeartWare LVAD. (*B*) The impeller of the pump is a centrifugal pump, suspended within the housing without any mechanical contact by magnets and a hydrodynamic thrust bearing. (*C*) The small pump, which is incorporated into the inflow sewing cuff, is placed in the pericardium with no need to create a pocket. (*Courtesy of* HeartWare Inc.)

device technology. One example is appropriate patient selection for the device therapy. Implantations performed in patients who have become too ill with multiorgan dysfunction, right ventricular dysfunction, functional impairment, and so on, have been consistently associated with adverse outcomes. Many scoring systems have been tested and advocated to improve patient selection1.[4,16] For the DT patient population, Lietz and colleagues[6] developed a risk score based on simple clinical parameters. The risk score was derived from the US population of mostly ambulatory DT recipients and intended to help estimate the probability of in-hospital death after elective LVAD surgery in patients who are not eligible for HTx. However, this score was developed based on the experience on HM VE and XVE, and may not be applicable to the CF LVAD patient population. Better outcome of LVAD therapy will parallel continuous efforts to seek better patient selection and postoperative care.

SUMMARY

LVAD therapy as DT has made a large leap with HM II technology, which is more reliable and durable. CF does not seem to have a detrimental effect on end-organ function, at least in the midterm. The smaller pump of the HM II with its axial flow mechanism is quieter than that of the HM XVE, and accessories, such as batteries and controller, are improved. These refinements have significantly contributed to a better quality of life for patients. The HM II will remain central to LVAD use for DT for the foreseeable future. However, many patients who have undergone HTx after being bridged with an HM II stated that their quality of life improved after transplantation (personal experience). More research is needed to further improve care of end-stage HF patients with LVAD technology.

REFERENCES

1. Rose EA, Gelijns AC, Moskowitz AJ, et al. Long-term mechanical left ventricular assistance for end-stage heart failure. N Engl J Med 2001;345(20):1435–43.
2. Slaughter MS, Rogers JG, Milano CA, et al. Advanced heart failure treated with continuous-flow left ventricular assist device. N Engl J Med 2009; 361(23):2241–51.
3. Rogers JG, Butler J, Lansman SL, et al. Chronic mechanical circulatory support for inotrope-dependent heart failure patients who are not transplant candidates: results of the INTrEPID Trial. J Am Coll Cardiol 2007;50(8):741–7.
4. Pae WE, Connell JM, Adelowo A, et al. Does total implantability reduce infection with the use of a left ventricular assist device? The LionHeart experience in Europe. J Heart Lung Transplant 2007;26(3): 219–29.
5. Dowling RD, Park SJ, Pagani FD, et al. HeartMate VE LVAS design enhancements and its impact on device reliability. Eur J Cardiothorac Surg 2004; 25(6):958–63.
6. Lietz K, Long JW, Kfoury AG, et al. Outcomes of left ventricular assist device implantation as destination therapy in the post-REMATCH era: implications for patient selection. Circulation 2007;116(5):497–505.
7. Farkas E, Elefteriades J. Assisted circulation: experience with the Novacor Left Ventricular Assist System. Expert Rev Med Devices 2007;4:769–74.
8. Kirklin JK, Naftel DC, Kormos RL, et al. Third INTERMACS Annual Report: the evolution of destination therapy in the United States. J Heart Lung Transplant 2011;30(2):115–23.
9. Kamdar F, Boyle A, Liao K, et al. Effects of centrifugal, axial, and pulsatile left ventricular assist device support on end-organ function in heart failure patients. J Heart Lung Transplant 2009;28(4):352–9.
10. Russell SD, Roger JG, Milano CA, et al. Renal and hepatic function improve in advanced heart failure patients during continuous-flow support with the HeartMate II left ventricular assist device. Circulation 2009;120:2352–7.
11. Petrucci RJ, Wright S, Naka Y, et al. Neurocognitive assessments in advanced heart failure patients receiving continuous-flow left ventricular assist devices. J Heart Lung Transplant 2009;28(6): 542–9.
12. Pak SW, Uriel N, Takayama H, et al. Prevalence of de novo aortic insufficiency during long-term support with left ventricular assist devices. J Heart Lung Transplant 2010;29(10):1172–6.
13. Cowger J, Pagani FD, Haft JW, et al. The development of aortic insufficiency in left ventricular assist device-supported patients. Circ Heart Fail 2010; 3(6):668–74.
14. Uriel N, Pak SW, Jorde UP, et al. Acquired von Willebrand syndrome after continuous-flow mechanical device support contributes to a high prevalence of bleeding during long-term support and at the time of transplantation. J Am Coll Cardiol 2010;56(15): 1207–13.
15. Rao V, Oz MC, Flannery MA, et al. Revised screening scale to predict survival after insertion of a left ventricular assist device. J Thorac Cardiovasc Surg 2003;125(4):855–62.
16. Gracin N, Johnson MR, Spokas D, et al. The use of APACHE II scores to select candidates for left ventricular assist device placement. Acute Physiology and Chronic Health Evaluation. J Heart Lung Transplant 1998;17(10):1017–23.

Editorial Comments on "Current Technology—Devices Available for 'Destination' Therapy"

John A. Elefteriades, MD

KEY CONCEPTS

Dr Yoshifumi Naka and colleagues provide a superb overview of traditional and newer devices for destination therapy in their article titled "Current Technology—Devices Available For 'Destination' Therapy." The investigators point out clearly that the theoretical concerns over potential damaging effects of nonpulsatile flow are simply not borne out.

STRENGTHS

Naka and colleagues detail the novel findings they have achieved regarding the continued incidence of stroke, continued incidence of bleeding, and curious induction of aortic insufficiency with continuous flow (CF) devices (HeartMate II).

WEAKNESSES

Experience with CF devices remains relatively short. Additional evidence will accumulate quickly through INTERMACS (Interagency Registry for Mechanically Assisted Circulatory Support).

Section of Cardiac Surgery, Yale University School of Medicine, Boardman 2, 333 Cedar Street, New Haven, CT 06510, USA
E-mail address: john.elefteriades@yale.edu

Cardiol Clin 29 (2011) 505
doi:10.1016/j.ccl.2011.07.005
0733-8651/11/$ – see front matter © 2011 Published by Elsevier Inc.

Avoiding Technical Pitfalls in Left Ventricular Assist Device Placement

John A. Elefteriades, MD[a],*, Donald M. Botta Jr, MD[b]

KEYWORDS

- Left ventricular assist device • Operative techniques
- Jarvik 2000 • Surgical pitfalls • LVAD • Hertmate II

Left ventricular assist device (LVAD) placement is a serious surgical procedure. At our center, we accumulated a large experience with the Novacor LVAD from the very first clinical trial, as well as from more recent experiences with the (Jarvik 2000, Jarvik Heart, New York, NY, USA) and the (HeartMate II, Thoratec Corporation, Pleasanton, CA, USA). This article discusses technical issues that are common to all LVAD devices, with special emphasis on strategy and technical considerations aimed at avoiding surgical pitfalls.

STERNOTOMY VERSUS LEFT THORACOTOMY

Placing the LVAD through a sternotomy has several disadvantages. The LVAD placement is often a reoperation, so all the dangers of sternal reentry are incurred. Furthermore, the subsequent heart transplant needs to be performed through a redo midsternotomy, with all the dangers of a second or third reentry. The outflow conduit of the LVAD to the ascending aorta is especially vulnerable; entry into the outflow graft can be catastrophic. The surgeon should be aware that cautery injuries to the graft can be impossible to control. The cautery can carry farther than the surgeon expects. The cautery tends to burn the graft in such a way that repair sutures do not hold well, and the cautery injury is usually at the limits of exposure, further impeding surgical control. Institution of cardiopulmonary bypass (CPB) is usually required.

All these issues can be avoided by placing the LVAD through a left thoracotomy. Left thoracotomy provides access via virgin territory. Furthermore, at a later date, when the transplant is being done through a sternotomy, this will again be via virgin territory, and there will be no vulnerable outflow conduit. These are dramatic advantages. We reported, many years ago, use of the Novacor LVAD via a left thoracotomy, with the outflow graft placed to the descending aorta (**Fig. 1**). The Jarvik 2000 is especially well suited to such an approach. When it is time for a transplant, the outflow graft is simply mobilized and transected after stapling with a vascular stapler. The other axial flow devices currently available are not designed or recommended for thoracotomy placement.

ON-PUMP OR OFF-PUMP PLACEMENT

Most LVADs are placed on CPB for multiple reasons. The patients are often unstable and need to be supported by CPB. With approach via sternotomy, the left ventricular (LV) apex needs to be elevated severely, which is not tolerated by these intrinsically compromised hearts. Many connectors are designed for deliberate placement into an open apical left ventriculotomy, with the heart supported on CPB and fibrillating.

The Jarvik 2000 is especially suited for placement without CPB. This finding was reported by Frazier, and we have used this approach with satisfaction. Via a left thoracotomy, the heart

[a] Section of Cardiac Surgery, Yale University School of Medicine, Boardman 2, 333 Cedar Street, New Haven, CT 06510, USA
[b] Cardiovascular Surgeons, P.A., 217 Hillcrest Street, Orlando, FL 32801, USA
* Corresponding author.
E-mail address: john.elefteriades@yale.edu

Cardiol Clin 29 (2011) 507–514
doi:10.1016/j.ccl.2011.08.008

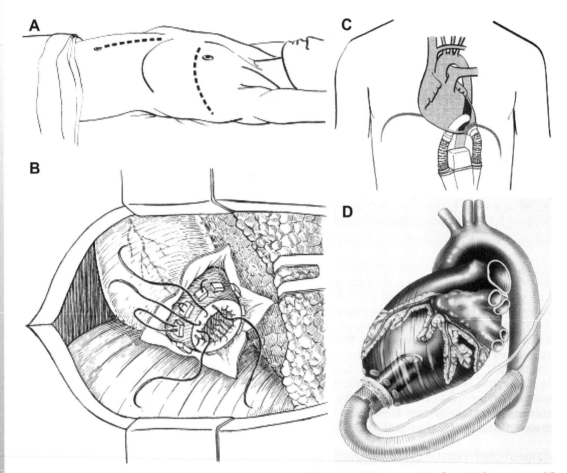

Fig. 1. Implantation of Novacor LVAD via left thoracotomy. (*A*) Incision. (*B*) Preparation for apical connector. (*C*) Final result (note outflow to descending aorta). (*D*) Left thoracotomy is also a preferred approach for Jarvik 2000.

does not need to be elevated or displaced at all to access the LV apex. Rather, the apex is right there. The descending aorta is readily accessible for anastomosis to the outflow conduit with a side-biting clamp. This is usually done first. The LV apical sutures are placed with the heart beating. There is usually little or no cardiac instability during these preparations. Then, the apex is cored with the coring device, the opening covered briefly with the thumb, and the Jarvik placed into the LV. There is a beauty and simplicity to this approach.

PROTECTION OF THE RIGHT VENTRICLE

When the LVAD is placed through a sternotomy on CPB, CPB is used during placement of LV apical sutures, coring of the apex, and placement of the apical connector. Cardioplegic arrest of the heart is unnecessary for any of these maneuvers, and it is usually avoided. It is important to remember, as pointed out by Akins many years ago, that the

right ventricle (RV) is vulnerable during fibrillatory arrest. Accordingly, we follow 2 precautions. First, we keep the perfusion pressure on the high side. Second, we make certain that the heart (LV and RV) remains nondistended at all times. In the setting of LVAD placement, this is easily and economically accomplished by coring the LV apex as soon as CPB is initiated, thus assuring decompression of the heart.

REENTRY FOR LVAD PLACEMENT

Many LVAD placements are done in patients who have had prior cardiac surgical procedures, including coronary artery bypass, aortic or mitral valve replacement, aortic aneurysm resection, or LV aneurysm resection. All issues of safe sternal division and heart chamber dissection and mobilization that apply to standard cardiac reoperations apply to LVAD operations as well. However, in patients with LVAD, some unique issues apply.

Importance of Computed Tomographic Scan

We routinely use a computed tomographic (CT) scan to show the relationship of the cardiac structures with the inner table of the sternum. We pay particular attention to the RV, which is likely chronically distented in a patient with heart failure. The relationship of the ascending aorta to the breastbone, as well as that of any vein or arterial grafts, is also assessed vis-à-vis vulnerability during reentry (**Fig. 2** A and B).

Venous Congestion

All systemic veins are likely to be engorged in a patient with heart failure severe enough to require LVAD placement. This engorgement should be anticipated during sternotomy and special care taken to achieve good hemostasis, especially of the veins in the suprasternal notch, sternal periosteum, and upper mediastinum.

RV Distension

It is likely, if not invariable, that the RV will be distended. This distention makes sternal division in redo operations especially hazardous. We advise having the femoral artery (and, perhaps, the femoral vein as well) exposed in advance of sternal division. In this way, CPB can be instituted quickly in case of RV injury during reentry.

Cardiac Enlargement

The LV, as well as the RV and both the atria, is likely to be significantly enlarged, making mobilization more challenging than in a non-LVAD case.

DISSECTION AND HEMOSTASIS

One of the strongest correlates with RV failure after LVAD placement is transfusion requirement. Patients with advanced heart failure are at particular risk for intraoperative and postoperative hemorrhage because most are coagulopathic going into the operating room. This coagulopathy can be caused by passive hepatic congestion from increased right atrial pressure or incomplete reversal of preoperative anticoagulant or antiplatelet agents. Postoperatively, these patients must be anticoagulated to prevent device thrombosis, and many experience bleeding due to platelet destruction, ongoing liver dysfunction, and acquired von Willebrand factor deficiency.

For this reason, all dissections must be meticulous and directed. No unnecessary dissection should occur. When hemodynamics allows, all dissections, including creation of ventricular assist device (VAD) pockets, driveline tunneling, chest tube incisions, placement of securing sutures, and dissection to allow for cannulation, should be performed before heparinization. The outflow conduit can be performed after giving an initial 5000-U heparin bolus, with full heparinization to follow.

When forming the driveline pocket in the preperitoneal space, we begin by placing a table-mounted retractor to elevate the left sternum and rectus abdominis sheath. Blunt dissection should be almost exclusively used, with targeted use of cautery. The left diaphragm should be divided

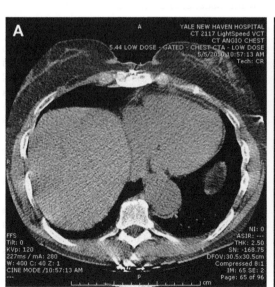
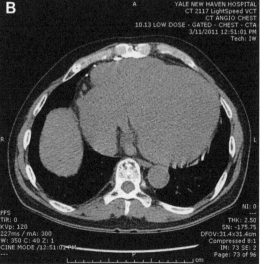

Fig. 2. (*A*) Good room is seen between the inner table of the sternum and the RV. (*B*) No space remains between the distended RV and the breastbone, a high-risk scenario.

with a gastrointestinal anastomosis (GIA)-type stapling device, which we have found yields much better hemostasis than division by cautery. Once the pocket is created, we loosely place a sponge in the pocket and remove the table-mounted retractor. After a pause, we remove the sponge and inspect once again for hemostasis, realizing that this is our final opportunity to have good visualization of this area.

In the case of the HeartMate II, we place both chest tubes and the pacing wires in the left rectus abdominis sheath, so as to reserve the right side for the driveline.

AIR

Air embolism is an important potential problem with any open cardiac surgical procedure, and each cardiac surgeon has his/her own techniques for its avoidance. In the case of LVAD placement, however, the potential problem of air embolism is especially acute. There are multiple reasons why air is especially important and dangerous in LVAD placement. The LV is wide open. Air can enter the arterial circulation from 2 routes. It can pass out the aortic valve through the native channel, or it can pass via the VAD into the ascending aorta. Also, as in any cardiac operation, the air is most likely to pass into the right coronary artery; this is especially dangerous because the RV is nearly always compromised and precarious in patients with LVAD. Air embolism to the right coronary artery on weaning CPB after LVAD placement produces acute and severe RV compromise, and recovery in such patients may be difficult or impossible. So, air takes on a much higher level of importance than in the average open cardiac surgical procedure.

So, we take several precautions. We flood the field with carbon dioxide (CO_2). As indicated in **Fig. 3**, CO_2 is heavier than atmospheric air and fills the pericardial well; so any air emboli will be CO_2-rich rather than nitrogen-rich atmospheric air. The CO_2 is resorbed much more rapidly and readily than nitrogen, leading to a very transient disruption of RV function in case of air embolism. We are careful to fill the LV well before attaching the apical connector. We deair both near the LV and in the outflow cannula proximal to the outflow anastomosis; we often use an aspirating needle connected to pump suction, as in our routine open cardiac cases. Also, as is standard in cardiac surgery, we use the Trendelenburg position to protect the brain.

Another time when air can be a problem is at the time of weaning from CPB. It must be assured that the heart is adequately filled (by decreasing the

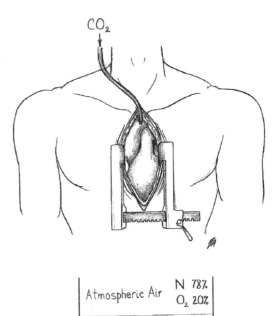

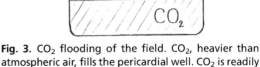

Fig. 3. CO_2 flooding of the field. CO_2, heavier than atmospheric air, fills the pericardial well. CO_2 is readily absorbed from any air emboli.

venous return to the heart-lung machine) so that air is not "sucked in" from around the apical connector or from other connections specific to each LVAD.

OUTFLOW ANASTOMOSIS

The end-to-side anastomosis of the outflow graft to the ascending aorta must be hemostatic. We recommend extreme care to incorporate both intima and adventitia in all bites. The side-biting clamp application must be generous enough to permit an adequate incision in the aorta and adequate visibility of the aortic edges for optimal construction of the anastomosis. We sometimes make only an incision and at other times take out a small ellipse of aortic wall, depending on the local circumstances. We recommend care in suturing around the heel and toe and also deliberate tightening of the suture line.

We usually perform the outflow anastomosis off pump but with the patient heparinized and cannulated. By doing this anastomosis off pump, we minimize CPB time. However, in some precarious patients, application of the side-biter may increase afterload enough to make the heart falter. We watch carefully the first few minutes for any decrease in arterial pressure or increase in filling pressure. If the heart does not tolerate the side-biter, we simply go on to CPB.

The length and lie of the outflow graft are critical. Too short a graft creates tension and bleeding. The graft should be long enough to lie to the right, so that the graft is not directly vulnerable during sternal reentry for transplantation. However, too long a graft may kink, causing failure of LVAD function.

LV APEX CONNECTION

Connecting to the LV apex is a serious endeavor not trivial in any way. Problems with this cannulation do occur and can be catastrophic.

Identification of the Apex

The apex can be identified both visually and by palpation. By palpation, it feels like a dimple when invaginated by the index finger. By inspection, the apex serves as a center point fulcrum for the counterclockwise rotation of the ventricular muscle; the apex is the point about which the heart muscle rotates.

The Distal Left Anterior Descending Coronary Artery

The left anterior descending (LAD) artery is very close to the apical sutures in the 9-o'clock region of the sewing ring. If on preoperative angiography the LAD is seen to terminate at the LV apex, it is acceptable to incorporate the distal LAD in the apical sutures. However, if there is a wraparound LAD (the "mermaid's tail") or if there is no preoperative angiography, the LAD should be deliberately spared by placing the apical sutures to the left of the LAD.

Sutures

Most surgeons use a set of deep mattress sutures placed circumferentially around the LV apex (using the apical sewing ring as a guide), with pledgets, and, occasionally, with a complete ring of Teflon felt. If these sutures are placed before the coring of the apex, it is important that they be placed deeply. If these sutures are placed after the ventriculotomy, they can be placed transmurally under direct vision, from epicardium to endocardium and then coming out from endocardium to epicardium. This placement produces an everting mattress suture. The inner outgoing endocardium to epicardium portion of the suture should incorporate only a thin (1–2 mm) portion of endocardium, myocardium, and epicardium. This prevents a bulky segment of myocardium from being forced into the apical opening when the sewing cuff is secured. Either the preapical or postapical coring method is acceptable. It is important that these sutures do not lacerate the myocardium as they are placed. Laceration is more likely to occur when they are placed on the beating heart before coring the apex under fibrillatory arrest. When these sutures are tied, it is imperative that they be tied tight enough to buckle the myocardial tissue but not tight enough that they tear the muscle itself.

On/Off Bypass

As explained previously, the sutures can be placed off bypass on the beating heart before coring the LV apex or on bypass, with the LV fibrillating to prevent ejection, either before or after LV coring. If the sutures are placed before bypass and coring, it is imperative to avoid cutting the sutures with the coring device when it is fired. It is not usually catastrophic if 1 or 2 sutures happen to be cut by the coring device; they can be replaced after the apical connector is seated and the intact sutures are tied. However, it is essential to make certain that none of the suture or pledget material is free to enter the LV cavity and can be ejected as an embolus.

Cutting Opening

Coring the LV apex is not trivial either. This procedure can be done free hand with a scalpel or a mechanical coring device. In either case, the apical connector should be a tight fit in the opening created.

Myocardial Debris (Doughnut)

When cutting the apical opening with the coring device, it is favorable to see a complete doughnut of material in the coring device after it is removed, signifying a complete cut, with no free pieces of myocardial debris. If this is not the case, the LV should be explored through the apex to ascertain that the opening is adequate and that no myocardial debris is free in the LV cavity. The LV should also be explored for thrombus at this point, and any loose chordate tendineae should be excised.

LV Apical Connector Angulation

It is important to insert the LV apical connector in an optimal direction and orientation. The connector should not abut the LV septal wall or the LV lateral wall. The connector should aim toward the mitral valve, so that it can collect the blood entering the LV optimally.

LV Apical Rotational Alignment

When placing a VAD through a sternotomy, the LV apex is rotated into the field for apical cannulation. Once the LV apex is allowed to return to its anatomic position, rotation of the sewing cuff about the axis of the apical cannula should be allowed to occur to avoid torsional stress about the LV apex. To accomplish this, we place the ligatures circumferentially around the sewing cuff but only loosely secure them with snares while the LV apex is in the operative field. Once the apical cannula is in place and the heart has returned to its anatomic position, we remove the snares and secure the ligatures tightly (we use 2 number 2 silks in addition to the green ligature that comes attached to the sewing cuff).

Bleeding from the LV Apex

Bleeding from the LV apex after placement of the apical connector can be catastrophic. It is best avoided by careful technique. Bleeding can be caused by indelicate suture placement, in which the needle tip is made to act like a blade instead of a needle, causing a linear radially oriented tear in the LV myocardium. This same linear radially oriented tear can occur from tying the apical sutures too tightly, again tearing the muscle tissue. The LV muscle can be torn during forceful placement of the apical connector, especially if the heart is perfused and beating or fibrillating and the opening is too small; a hypertrophied LV can seem as if it is contracting like a sphincter when the surgeon attempts to place the apical connector. Further incision of the opening or gentle dilatation with a finger or dilator is indicated. The LV apex can also tear when the heart is replaced in the resting position from the elevated position used during suture placement and connector insertion; the connector is rigid and the muscle is delicate. Also, in some cases, the tissue is so friable that tearing can occur even with the most delicate optimal technique. Bleeding from the apex usually requires placement of additional sutures. These sutures should be large, incorporating a good amount of muscle tissue, and supported by generous pledgets. In the case of a linear radially oriented tear, the sutures can be placed perpendicular to the tear, that is, tangential to the sewing ring. In most instances, however, the repair sutures are placed similar to the original apical sutures, radially from peripheral to central, into the sewing ring. We tend to use a trick we learned doing LV resections with Dr Batista in Brazil. We incorporate a large piece of autologous fat into the large mattress sutures used for repair in case of LV apical bleeding (**Fig. 4**). The fatty tissue makes an excellent plug for the bleeding site. This technique can be literally lifesaving. We sometimes "tan" some fatty tissue in advance with glutaraldehyde and keep it ready in case needed for this technique.

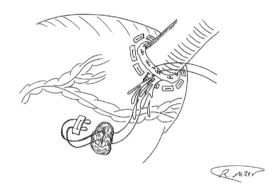

Fig. 4. Use of a (glutaraldehyde treated) fat pad as a pledget to control bleeding from an LV apex cannulated for LVAD. The fat exerts an excellent and durable tamponade effect, like having one's finger in place permanently.

LVAD DRIVELINE

Issues regarding the LVAD driveline are covered fully in the driveline article by Dr Conte and colleagues in this issue.

LVAD POCKET

With the (HeartMate XV, Thoratec Corporation, Pleasanton, CA, USA), and especially the Novacor, large pockets were required for placement of the device. These pockets were cumbersome to develop, often served as sites of bleeding, and constituted fertile ground for closed-space pocket infections. Fortunately, the newer continuous flow devices have low to minimal space needs. The Jarvik 2000 fits entirely within the LV and needs no pocket. The HeartMate II does need some room for the pump to "sit" after the heart is returned from the elevated position.

THE HEARTMATE "SLING"

A very useful technique for dividing the diaphragm, protecting the abdominal contents and minimizing subsequent adhesions when forming a pocket for the HeartMate II, is to create a sling using expanded polytetrafluoroethylene (Gore-Tex) (**Fig. 5**). A cone is formed by cutting an isosceles triangle out of Gore-Tex at approximately 15 cm in the long axis and 10 cm in the short axis. Depending on the size of the patient and the distance from the midline to the chest wall, the length dimension should be adjusted. This triangle is formed into a cone by suturing the free edges together with 5-0 Prolene. The cone is placed into the preperitoneal space with the

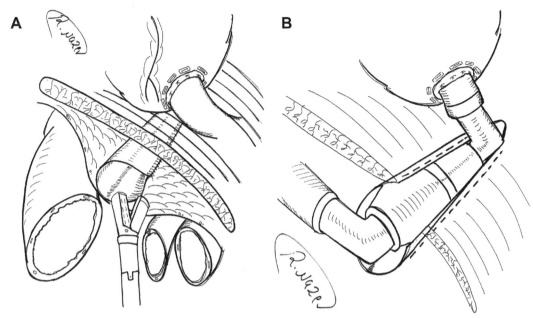

Fig. 5. (*A, B*) The HeartMate sling.

Prolene abutting the intact diaphragm and the sharp end abutting the chest wall. An endo-GIA stapling device (green load) is then placed onto the Prolene suture line, incorporating both the cone and the diaphragm, and fired. Firings of the stapling device are repeated until the apex of the cone is reached.

BLEEDING

As discussed previously, bleeding can be problematic after LVAD placement for many reasons: preexisting clotting abnormalities due to congestive heart failure and liver dysfunction, high venous pressures (occasional), long pump times, multiple ventricular and aortic suture lines, and other reasons. If cardiac output and pump function are suffering, in a patient previously doing well, bleeding should be suspected to have caused a local tamponade effect that impairs filling of the LVAD. Although cardiac echocardiography can be useful, the windows of transthoracic echocardiography are notoriously poor, especially in the area of the lateral and superior portion of the right atrium and the proximal aorta, where blood and thrombus commonly collect after LVAD placement. Surgeons placing VAD should have a very low threshold for reexploration. In addition, reexploration for bleeding should not be used as a quality measure in VAD programs for 2 reasons: (1) the need for reexploration is common and more often dependent on patient factors than surgical technique and (2) the decision to reexplore is a difficult one and should not be influenced by administrative factors.

We recommend the following measures to minimize the likelihood of bleeding.

Advance Factors

Because so many patients have preexisting hepatic dysfunction and coagulopathy, we pretreat those with these conditions with vitamin K (10 mg intravenously) to optimize the native coagulation cascade. We also recommend early cessation of anticoagulant and antiplatelet agents.

Aprotinin was wonderful for such cases, until its withdrawal; aprotinin produced a perfectly dry field after major aortic and LVAD surgery. In its absence, factor VII is becoming more popular. Routine administration of factor VII is worth considering in LVAD cases. We use one-third to one-half the recommended dose, in the range of 3 to 5 mg. We have occasionally encountered untoward thrombosis with the full dose of factor VII or with repeat doses.

Glues

We are not above application of glues to the aortic suture line and the apical connection. A variety of effective topical agents are available.

Care with Anticoagulation

We recommend discretion in starting anticoagulants after LVAD placement. The situation usually produces considerable coagulopathy by its very nature. We wait until the patient is perfectly dry before starting anticoagulants. Depending on the device, we usually avoid postoperative heparin altogether, starting warfarin sodium (Coumadin) and antiplatelet drugs late on the day of or early on the day after LVAD placement. It is important to remember that a patient with a graft to aorta anastomosis, if given heparin uninterrupted from the time of surgery onward, will be extremely prone to exsanguinating hemorrhage; after all, the spaces between sutures are sealed by thrombus. We recommend discretion in heparin administration in this setting.

Practical tips for LVAD placement are summarized in **Box 1**.

Box 1
Practical tips for LVAD placement

Remember the left thoracotomy approach, it has many advantages at the time of placement and time of transplant.

Remember the option of off-pump placement of the LVAD, it is elegantly simple.

Remember to protect the RV while on CPB. Keep the heart empty and the perfusion pressure high.

Use great caution during reentry for LVAD placement. The distended RV will be especially vulnerable, as will be the ascending aorta and any vein or arterial grafts.

Use a preoperative CT scan to assess and localize sites of reentry vulnerability/safety.

Place the sternal retractor upside down, with the ratchet mechanism in a cephalad direction.

Air is your enemy:

> The vulnerable, chronically straining RV will not tolerate air embolism to the right coronary artery on weaning CPB.

> Use CO_2 flooding of the field.

> Fill the LV before attaching the apical connector.

> Be sure that the heart is adequately filled on weaning CPB, so as to not "suck" air.

> Remember that air can egress the heart through both the native LV and aortic valve as well as through the LVAD to the ascending aorta.

> Use a continuous needle to pump suction to protect the brain.

For the outflow anastomosis to the ascending aorta, it is imperative to use care at the heel and toe areas and to tighten the suture line deliberately.

Length and lie of the outflow graft are critical to prevent tension, prevent kinking (with consequent LVAD failure), and keep the graft out of harm's way during sternal reentry for transplantation.

When the LV apex sutures are tied, it is imperative that they be tied tight enough to buckle the myocardial tissue but not tight enough that they tear the muscle itself.

In coring the LV apex, be on alert for cut apical sutures, an incomplete doughnut of apical resected tissue, and stray pieces of cut myocardial debris, which can be embolized systemically when cardiac activity resumes.

It is OK to incorporate the terminal LAD in the apical sutures as a sort of autologous pledget if the LAD terminates at the cardiac apex.

In case of LV apex myocardial bleeding, a large piece of the patient's own fatty tissue can be used as a plug within the mattress sutures used for repair.

The GIA stapler (often with a Gore-Tex membrane) can automatically cut and control the periapex diaphragm, making a comfortable easy pocket for the HeartMate II (and similar devices) to lie when the heart is replaced in its native position.

To prevent bleeding, administer vitamin K in advance, use topical glues on the anastomoses, wait until the patient is "dry" to anticoagulate, and use extreme discretion with continuous intravenous heparin.

Left Ventricular Assist Device Driveline Infections

Daniel Pereda, MD, John V. Conte, MD*

KEYWORDS

• Left ventricular assist device • Heart failure • Infection

GENERAL OVERVIEW

Left ventricular assist devices (LVADs) represent one of the major advances in the modern management of patients with end-stage heart failure, and have been shown to provide longer survival and better quality of life in these patients in comparison with optimal medical therapy.[1] Although the initial attention was focused on their use in bridging patients awaiting heart transplantation, the higher survival rates observed among LVAD recipients together with the limited availability of organ donors have expanded their use as destination therapy as well.[2] However, and despite all the technical advances in their design and the improvement in postoperative management of these patients, LVAD therapy is still associated with some important complications, among which the following stand out: hemorrhagic and thromboembolic events, device failure, arrhythmias, and infection. In recent years an important shift has occurred in clinical LVAD use toward longer periods of mechanical support before recovery or transplantation, corresponding to the more recently approved indication as destination therapy in patients who are not candidates for heart transplantation. This trend increases even more the relevance of these problems, because most of them are cumulative over time and, therefore, their prevalence increases as duration of support lengthens.

Although continuous advance in LVAD design and technology have contributed to reducing most of these risks compared with previous models, infection continues to be one of the most prevalent problems, with major clinical and economic consequences. All of the LVAD components are susceptible to infection, each with their own specific characteristics and clinical implications. On the one hand, infection of the internal blood-contacting surfaces of the pump or of the inflow and outflow grafts represents an intravascular infection, a situation similar to endocarditis. On the other hand, infection located on the external surface of the device and its surrounding pocket, including the percutaneous driveline internal track and exit site, represents a completely different clinical scenario.

LVAD infections can originate through several different mechanisms, including microbial contamination during the implant procedure, progression of pathogens following the driveline path from the exit site in the skin, or hematogenous dissemination of organisms from an infection originating at a distant site with secondary involvement of the LVAD. Regardless of the source of the infection, early diagnosis is often not made and adequate treatment is subsequently delayed, which complicates the problem even further, often allowing extension of the infection to other LVAD components and deeper into the patient's tissues. This delay in correct diagnosis and treatment frequently leads to a situation requiring prolonged intravenous antibiotic therapy and aggressive surgical measures, such as extensive debridement, use of muscular or omental flaps, institution of chronic pump pocket irrigation-drainage systems, and even LVAD exchange.

As already outlined, in its early days LVAD therapy was designed to support patients for

The authors have nothing to disclose.
Division of Cardiac Surgery, Department of Surgery, Johns Hopkins Cardiac Surgery, The Johns Hopkins Medical Institutions, 600 North Wolfe Street, Blalock 618, Baltimore, MD 21287, USA
* Corresponding author.
E-mail address: jconte@jhmi.edu

Cardiol Clin 29 (2011) 515–527
doi:10.1016/j.ccl.2011.08.004
0733-8651/11/$ – see front matter

relatively short periods of time, always in an inpatient setting. Accordingly, the principal interest was placed on infections that occurred early in the course of LVAD therapy, and the advances made in the field have successfully addressed some of the problems with early infection. In fact, at present only about 15% of local infections occur during the first 30 days after LVAD implantation.[3] After the more recent paradigm shift that has occurred in LVAD therapy toward longer support and use as destination therapy, as well as increased patient autonomy and management in an outpatient setting, late device-related infections have been the main focus of interest.

Regardless of its origin and which LVAD component is involved, LVAD infection is a serious complication that can be life threatening. In the landmark REMATCH trial,[1] infections accounted for 41% of the deaths observed in patients on mechanical LVAD support. Survival analysis showed a 48% reduction in mortality from any cause after the first year in patients allocated to LVAD therapy. After 2 years, however, the survival rate of 23% was not statistically significant between the two groups. These data highlight the importance of prevention and management of LVAD infections and bacteremia to improve and extend the survival benefit in LVAD patients, especially beyond the first year. A study on bloodstream infections in patients bridged to transplantation showed an incidence of 7.9 bloodstream infections per 1000 LVAD days. Of these, 38% were related to the device, and other sources included: catheters (16%), respiratory infections (6%), abdominal infections (6%), urinary tract infections (1%), and unknown (29%).[4] Mortality was highest for fungal infections, followed by gram-negative bacilli and gram-positive cocci infections.

In addition to the life threatening risk that LVAD infections represent for patients, their management usually requires extended and repeated hospitalizations and intense outpatient care. LVAD-related infections ultimately endanger the final objectives of LVAD therapy, eliminating the intended patient autonomy, jeopardizing a possible heart transplant in patients bridged with this intention, and decreasing overall survival and quality of life.

Another important aspect to consider when discussing the effects of infection in these patients is the impact on costs of LVAD therapy. A subanalysis study[5] from the REMATCH trial data found that the principal drivers of implantation costs were sepsis, pump housing infection, and perioperative bleeding. In patients who did not present any of these complications, implantation cost was estimated at $119,874 By contrast, if only sepsis was present the cost rose to $263,822 and, if all

3 complications (sepsis, pump infection, perioperative bleeding) were present, the cost increased to $869,199. The device used in this trial was the HeartMate VE (Thoratec Corp, Pleasanton, CA) and its calculated cost was $60,000. This study also determined that the average cost of readmission for these patients was $30,627 ± $61,569 per readmission, and the average cost of readmissions during the first year of mechanical support in the whole LVAD cohort was $105,326 per patient.[5] In addition, another study has shown that the occurrence of late infections after successful LVAD implantation and initial discharge from the hospital increases significantly the number of readmissions per patient (from 0.5 ± 0.9 to 6 ± 4.8; $P<.001$) and the average duration in days of each readmission (from 1.8 ± 0.8 to 41.8 ± 26.8; $P<.001$).[3]

It seems clear that prevention of infections must become a central objective for hospital teams involved in the care of patients undergoing LVAD therapy. In this regard, preventive measures should start even before the moment of LVAD implantation and continue throughout the complete duration of mechanical support.

DRIVELINE INFECTION

The focus of LVAD infections has progressively shifted from the perioperative period toward late-onset infections. Among those infections appearing later after implantation, the most prevalent and important is infection of the LVAD driveline. In fact this has become the real Achilles' heel of long-term LVAD therapy with the present devices available in clinical practice. All continuous-flow LVADs currently in clinical use require this component (driveline) to deliver energy to the pump from the external energy source. The driveline also allows communication between the pump and the controller unit, exchanging telemetry data and algorithms that allow monitoring of the device function and changes in its operational settings.

In the pathogenesis of driveline infections, the presence of foreign material plays a major role. It is known that the existence of a foreign body enhances germ pathogenicity and impairs the host's immune response. In classic studies from the 1950s, it was shown that just the presence of a braided silk suture in the subcutaneous tissue remarkably facilitated infection, needing only the inoculation of 100 CFU of *Staphylococcus pyogenes* to cause a clinical infection, as compared with the 10^6 CFU needed when no foreign material was present.[6] Microorganisms can colonize the surface of foreign material at any time during or after implantation, and these colonies may remain silent for a long period of time, being able to produce clinically unconcealed infections months or even years after the original LVAD implantation.[7]

Definite diagnosis of percutaneous entry site or pump pocket infections usually requires a positive culture, obtained from the skin or tissue surrounding the driveline or from the tissue or fluid surrounding the external housing of the pump. Therapy requires antibiotic administration when clinical evidence of infection exists, such as fever, leukocytosis, or pain or drainage around the driveline entry site or its internal pathway.[8]

The main pathogenetic mechanisms of infection in LVAD patients after the perioperative period are largely linked to the LVAD driveline. This percutaneous channel acts as the port of entry for external pathogens, which can then migrate deeper through this tunnel into the host's tissues. If this process is not stopped, pathogens can even arrive at the pump itself, causing pocket infection, which may be extremely difficult to eradicate or even to control. In a recent study in patients receiving a HeartMate II device (Thoratec Corp) implanted as a bridge to transplant, there was a trend for slightly lower survival at 1 year after heart transplantation in patients who developed driveline infections during LVAD support when compared with those who had no infections (75% vs 89%; $P = .07$).[9] In this study the incidence of driveline infection was 17.5%, with a median duration of mechanical support of 151 days. Another previous study showed that in the bridge-to-transplant population, a positive driveline culture was found in 50% of patients successfully bridged at the moment of their heart transplant, and 30% had a clinically active infection.[10,11] In the population awaiting heart transplantation while on LVAD support, late infection was the reason for declining an organ in about 30% of cases.[11,12] Among patients who die of infection during LVAD support while awaiting transplantation, 29% had a driveline infection.[11,12]

Once the pump pocket is infected, patients are best managed by pump explant or heart transplantation,[13,14] interventions that carry a high risk of serious morbidity and mortality. Pump explant is more often needed when infection is caused by yeast or multidrug-resistant gram-negative bacilli.[15] Patients with complicated driveline infections, and especially those with pocket infections who are awaiting transplantation, may require upgrade to 1a status.

Epidemiology

Percutaneous drivelines remain a major source of infectious complications in patients supported with LVAD (**Table 1**). In a subanalysis of data

from the REMATCH trial, the prevalence of driveline or pocket infection was 28%, with an incidence of 0.36 cases per patient-year.[16] In the more recent trial with the HeartMate II device implanted as a bridge to transplant, the prevalence of driveline infection at 1 year was 14%, with an event rate of 0.37 cases per patient-year and no cases of pump pocket infection.[17]

Driveline infection is clearly related to the duration of mechanical support. In their study with the HeartMate I (Thoratec Corp) and the Novacor (World Heart Corp, Ottawa, ON, Canada) devices, Zierer and colleagues[3] described that the cumulative hazard for the development of a driveline infection increased dramatically with the duration of support, and calculated that the individual risk for developing a driveline infection after 1 year of LVAD support was 94%. Driveline infection was found in 23% of their patients after LVAD implant, appearing at a median of 158 days postimplant, and was attributed to driveline trauma in 77% of cases.[3] Of interest, in their 10-year study this tendency did not change in their more recent implants.[3] Another recent case-control study, among 118 patients undergoing mechanical support for at least 90 days (average 445 days), the incidence of driveline infection was 30%. In this study the mean duration of LVAD support among patients who had a driveline infection was 700 days, compared with 300 days for patients in the noninfected control group,[18] showing the cumulative nature of driveline infection and its relationship with duration of mechanical support.

Etiology and Pathogenesis

The most frequent microorganism implicated with LVAD driveline infections is *Staphylococcus epidermidis*.[19] Other microorganisms usually involved are *Staphylococcus aureus*, *Enterococcus* spp, *Corynebacterium* spp (*jejuni*), *Candida* spp, *Escherichia coli*, *Enterobacter faecalis*, *Klebsiella pneumoniae*, and *Pseudomonas aeruginosa*. LVAD Infections caused by *Candida* spp are associated with the highest mortality rate.[19,20]

LVAD driveline infection and progression into deeper structures is a complex multistep process produced by a large number of interrelated aspects that can be summarized and classified as follows: host determinants, microbiological determinants, implant and postoperative care determinants, and characteristics of the device itself. All these factors are interrelated, and all play a role in the origin and course of LVAD driveline infections.

Host determinants

Many characteristics related to patient basal characteristics, functional status, and comorbidities

Table 1
Incidence of infection in patients with left ventricular assist devices[a]

Authors[Ref.]	Year	Patients	Devices Used	Driveline Infection (%)	Other Infections	Mean Duration of Support (Days)	Median Time to Infection (Days)
Martin et al[59]	2010	145	MateMate I HeartMate II Thoratec IVAD VentrAssist Abiomed MicroMed	37	Bacteremia 41% Pocket 10% Sternal wound 12%	—	50
Holman et al[60]	2010	593	Only pulsatile	21	Bacteremia 32%	—	—
Aslam et al[61]	2010	300	HeartMate I HeartMate II Thoratec IVAD Jarvik2000	16	Bacteremia 19% Pocket 11% Endocarditis 6%	—	—
Saito et al[62]	2010	106	Toyobo HeartMate I Novacor Jarvik2000 EvaHeart DuraHeart	34	Bacteremia 43% Mediastinitis/ Pocket 15%	591	—
Pagani et al[63]	2009	281	HeartMate II	14	Sepsis 17% Pocket 2%	182	—
Morshuis et al[64]	2009	68	DuraHeart	15	Sepsis 18% Pocket 3%	242	—
Pae et al[65]	2007	23	LionHeart	Not available	Sepsis 30% Pocket 35%	347	—
Miller et al[17]	2007	133	HeartMate II	14	Sepsis 20% Pocket 0%	168	—
Monkowski et al[66]	2007	60	HeartMate I Thoratec	48	Endocarditis 22% Mediastinitis 5% Pocket 42%	159	150 d for driveline 90 d for pocket 80 d for endocarditis
Holman et al[16]	2004	68	HeartMate I	28	Sepsis 41% Pocket 16%	408	—

[a] This table is not meant to represent a systematic review of the available literature, only an example of recent data on this issue representative of different geographic areas and device options for mechanical ventricular support.

have an influence in the susceptibility to suffer infections after LVAD implantation. Among these factors the authors consider of special relevance patient nutritional status, immunosuppression (including preoperative medications), oral hygiene, diabetes, renal failure, and other comorbid conditions. Obesity has been related to a higher risk for driveline infection, which tends to appear earlier after implant in these patients.[18]

The need for frequent hospital admissions prior to the LVAD implant or a prolonged preoperative hospital admission are risk factors for LVAD infection. The preoperative presence of mechanical ventilation, vascular and urinary catheters, skin breakdown, nosocomial infections, and treatments with antimicrobial agents is frequent in such patients, serving as relevant risk factors for the appearance of postoperative infections in general and those caused by multidrug-resistant pathogens in particular.

Physical activity after LVAD implantation without the appropriate precautions to immobilize the driveline may cause important torque at the exit site. Shearing traction and rotation are the two mechanisms of injury at this location. Dropping the battery pack, moving without picking up the controller, or hooking the driveline on a passing object have been described as typical causes of serious damage to the driveline exit site. Excessive physical activity without adequate preventive measures to avoid driveline mobility produces continuous trauma around the exit site and leads to neoepithelialization, which further impedes adherence and facilitates microbial colonization. It has been shown that driveline infection is frequently preceded by deficient healing of the exit site.[21] The longer the duration of mechanical support, the more important this problem becomes, being of particular significance for patients on destination therapy.

Surgical implant and postoperative care determinants

Depurate surgical technique and meticulous postoperative care are essential in avoiding most postoperative complications, and particularly infections, after any surgical procedure. This fact is especially true for LVAD implantation procedures, given that patients receiving this treatment are usually in very poor condition and surgery involves implantation of a large foreign body, in direct and permanent communication with the exterior through the skin. The surgeon must take particular care in achieving good hemostasis during the implantation and assuring excellent drainage of all surgical sites, particularly the pump pocket, to evacuate all blood and fluids that may accumulate during the early postoperative period. Patients receiving an LVAD are at higher risk for postoperative bleeding compared with other cardiac procedures, and dissection performed to create the space needed to host the internal portion of the device may produce excessive fluid secretion, further stimulated by the presence of the device itself. Drains may need to remain in place for long periods of time after the implantation in many patients, until this production of fluid is reduced to a minimum and it is safe to remove them. Localized hematomas or fluid accumulation in the pump pocket can be colonized by bacteria and may become the source of infections late after the procedure. Another critical aspect of surgical technique is achieving a firm seal around the driveline exit site.[22] Immediately after surgery, the patient's tissues and microorganisms vie to establish domain over the surface of the implant. Good tissue integration onto the surface of the driveline is the best defense of the host against late-onset infection.[23] Purse-string sutures are usually placed around the exit site through the skin and must remain in place until the skin is completely and tightly healed around the driveline, a process that can take up to 30 days in some patients.[24]

Pump characteristics

The LVAD drivelines are coated in most models with a layer of highly textured polyester material that facilitates its integration into the skin and soft tissues, therefore protecting against bacterial entry through the exit site. The thicker and stiffer this driveline is, the higher the risk of trauma at the entry site and bacterial colonization. From initial LVAD designs, many advances have appeared to improve this situation. One of the first improvements made to reduce the risk of infection was moving from designs with multiple transcutaneous accesses to pumps that use only one larger single-lead driveline.[25] The newer continuous-flow LVADs, using drivelines with smaller diameters and increased flexibility, seem to reduce the incidence of driveline infections during mid-term follow-up.[26–28] The experience with these newer designs in terms of number of patients and duration of mechanical support is more limited than that available from earlier series using previous models, and many of these trends and hopes are awaiting confirmation.

Advances reducing the volume and weight of battery packs and controller units have the potential to decrease the incidence of driveline infections by reducing torque and tension at the exit site. This improvement will also allow patients on LVAD support enhanced mobility in safer conditions than with the currently available models.

Another field of ongoing research is the coating of the driveline and pump surfaces with antibiotic and antiseptic substances (as has been done with success on intravenous lines).[29] With this same rationale, the use of polymethylmethacrylate beads containing antibiotics such as tobramycin and vancomycin to coat the external surface of the pump has been also tested in patients bridged to transplant, in a way comparable with use in orthopedic surgery.[30]

In addition, several studies involving new strategies to avoid penetration of the flexible skin and subcutaneous tissue by the thick and stiff driveline structure are under development. One strategy involves fixation of the exit site to the skull,[21,31] in a similar way to cochlear implants. Another approach aims at discouraging epithelial downgrowth along the driveline by precoating the driveline surface with autologous fibroblasts cultured from a skin sample of the recipient (Viaderm percutaneous access device), and is being tested as part of the Kantrowitz CardioVad device study.[32] Finally, the development of transcutaneous energy delivery systems to completely avoid the necessity of the driveline at all[33–35] has, in the authors' view, the potential to completely overcome this problem (see the article by Bonde elsewhere in this issue). However, the technology needed to have a functionally efficient device using this approach is still not available.

Microbiological determinants

The key step in the initiation of the infection process is bacterial colonization of the exit site and the driveline surface. Staphylococci, such as S aureus and S epidermidis, possess a wide variety of surface proteins with versatile and redundant adhesive properties, many of them belonging to a structurally related family of microbial surface components recognizing adhesive matrix molecules (MSCRAMMs).[36] These proteins facilitate the initial colonization step, allowing the bacteria to start progressing centripetally along the driveline into deeper tissues, and even reaching the pump pocket. These and other microbiological features are now described in detail.

Pathogenesis

Driveline infection is a complex multistep process that usually originates around the exit site across the patient's skin. The exit site of the driveline is accessible to commensal flora present in the skin, and is exposed to repeated trauma directly related to driveline mobilization that impairs integration of the host's tissue into the surface of the driveline.[37] Maintaining a healthy exit site is important because the damaged tissues expose fibronectin, fibrin,

and platelets, facilitating bacterial adhesion. Some bacteria commonly present in the skin possess an intrinsic ability to adhere and colonize both the skin and the device surface, establishing the driveline exit site as the portal of entry for more serious infections of the device components.[38,39] Immediately after implantation, all foreign surfaces of the implanted LVAD and its driveline begin to acquire a biofilm containing fibronectin, fibrin, collagen, lipids, and inorganic ions. Collagen has been shown to be the major component that coats the surface of the internal driveline, which is also covered by cellular elements such as fibroblasts and myofibroblasts.[38] This process creates a matrix to which microorganisms can easily attach.[40–43] Colonizing microorganisms have specific and nonspecific receptors on their surface able to interact with and attach to the bare foreign material and to this biofilm. This biofilm also seems to facilitate migration of microorganisms along the driveline, progressing deeper into the host's tissues and allowing infection to spread to other organs.[44] Bacteria then start producing a protective exopolysaccharide layer, known as "slime," that entraps circulating nutrients and provides a mechanical defensive barrier against both humoral[41–43] and cellular[45] immune responses from the host. This slime barrier has also been shown to decrease the efficiency of antibiotic treatments[46] up to 500-fold.[47]

In addition to these important local components, several systemic factors have been related to the pathogenesis of infections in patients with LVAD. Some specific immunologic changes seem to occur after the implantation of an LVAD, and have raised the interest of investigators because they may play a role in susceptibility to infections and the ability of the host to effectively fight them. Several studies have demonstrated a reduced proliferative lymphocyte capacity in peripheral blood after the implantation of an LVAD. This reduction might be produced by the immune response of the host against the device, and it has been suggested that it eventually leads to local and systemic immunocompromise.[48,49]

The presence of the LVAD may produce an aberrant activation of T cells that finally results in cell apoptosis. These defects in cellular immune response could place patients at increased risk of infections by Candida spp.[48] In addition to this impairment in cellular immune response, patients with LVADs also show cytokine production imbalance. Specifically, the expression of proinflammatory cytokines interleukin (IL)-2 and tumor necrosis factor α is reduced, and IL-10 expression is elevated in CD3[+] T cells compared with patients with advanced chronic heart failure but without

LVAD support.[50] The humoral immune response is also impaired, and up to 23% of patients under LVAD support show hypogammaglobulinemia.[51] The reason for this is not completely understood and is probably multifactorial. However, hypogammaglobulinemia seems to be related to an increased susceptibility to major infections and bacteremia during mechanical support, in comparison with patients with normal IgG levels and also with a higher risk for cytomegalovirus infection after heart transplantation.[51]

Prevention

As previously discussed, prevention is the most efficient element against infections in patients with LVADs. Preventive measures to avoid driveline infection must begin as soon as possible, even before LVAD implantation, with optimization of the recipient's nutritional status and avoidance of implantation in already colonized or infected recipients, particularly when microorganisms with the potential to generate infection of the device are involved. Antibiotic prophylaxis before implantation is mandatory, and the recommended duration of the prophylactic antibiotic treatment usually extends 24 to 48 hours after the procedure. It is thought that extending the prophylactic coverage does not reduce the infection rate further, and may actually increase the risk of selecting resistant pathogens. The antibiotic should be completely infused within 1 hour of skin incision to maximize the benefit. Intraoperative bleeding of greater than 1.5 L or procedure time extending beyond 2.5 times the half-life of the prophylactic agents used may require antibiotic redosing.[52] There might be a role for nasal decolonization in avoiding infections by gram-positive cocci, and routine surveillance cultures to assess S aureus carrier status are recommended. The protocol for antibiotic prophylaxis used by the authors in these patients has been previously reported,[53] and consists of a combination of vancomycin (1 g), ciprofloxacin (400 mg), and fluconazole (400 mg) dosed within 30 minutes of skin incision. Medications are redosed during the operation based on their pharmacokinetic properties. Antibiotic prophylaxis is continued until 48 hours after sternal closure using vancomycin (1 g every 12 hours), ciprofloxacin (400 mg every 12 hours), and fluconazole (400 mg every 24 hours), with adequate renal adjustment.

All measures to prevent contamination of the device or wound during the procedure must be adopted and all the staff in the operating room should follow strict infection control standards, limiting the number of people inside the room and reducing transit in and out of the room to the minimum needed.

As already mentioned, depurated surgical technique and postoperative care are also essential. One important aspect in avoiding driveline infections later after implantation is the selection of the optimal exit site location. Some of the factors to consider in this decision include patient body habitus and expected body weight changes, clothing lines, and anticipation of the impact of changing body position in the driveline. Care must be taken to prevent opening the peritoneal cavity during implantation because ascitic fluid may form collections around the pump in the pocket and in the driveline pathway, and its persistent drainage through the exit site impairs healing around the driveline. The exit site must be created by a small, clean stab wound in the skin (of about 75% of the driveline diameter) to keep a tight seal around the driveline, using a device designed specifically for this purpose.[3] Use of the cautery should be avoided, if possible, to prevent burns in the skin around the exit site. All surgical wounds must be closed without tension,[54] and complete immobilization of the driveline at the exit site must be accomplished. To achieve this, the driveline is sutured to the skin and retained immobile using drain-attachment devices or abdominal binders.

During the postoperative period, bacteremia must be avoided. Particular care must be observed in the placement and management of central lines. A depurated technique, adequate hand washing, barrier measures, and adequate prepping and site dressing are critical for this objective. The use of antiseptic-coated or antibiotic-coated intravenous lines may be helpful, particularly in patients receiving parenteral nutrition. During the postoperative period one should ensure good nutrition for the patient and avoid hyperglycemia.

One of the most critical aspects for prevention of driveline-related infections is exit site and driveline management. Careful sterile management of the exit site is of paramount importance. Daily antiseptic cures in a sterile fashion using hydrogen peroxide, povidone-iodine, or chlorhexidine solutions with sterile dressing changes should start 72 hours postoperatively, or sooner if dressings are saturated. Scheduled cures should follow once or twice daily thereafter. Routine dressing changes after discharge from hospital are started in the outpatient clinic, and once patients and families have been adequately instructed they are allowed to perform them at home on a weekly basis.

Wound irritation is usually caused by excess moisture at the exit site. Maceration can be treated by increasing the frequency of dressing changes.

While in the hospital dressing changes should be performed in a sterile fashion, and hospital staff doing them should have proper training and must wear a mask, gown, and cap. Customized dressing-change kits for inpatient use may be helpful in standardizing nursing care. All wounds must be inspected daily for the presence of early signs of impaired healing or infection so that appropriate measures can be rapidly adopted. There has been some interest in the use of silver-impregnated dressings, but data are lacking for their use at driveline exit sites.

Together with adequate in-hospital care, patients and caregivers must be educated and instructed in how to perform these tasks after hospital discharge and how to avoid activities that predispose to driveline trauma. Showering should be avoided during the first 30 days after implant and until adequate tissue ingrowth into the percutaneous tube velour has occurred, with no drainage or signs of infection at the exit site.

Diagnosis

One of the most important factors in combating driveline infections is early identification so as to allow aggressive treatment in the early stages. Several classification systems are available to grade the severity of driveline infections (**Box 1**). It is the authors' protocol to routinely obtain blood cultures on the first postoperative day, and then to send additional cultures on clinical suspicion of infection, acute neutropenia or leukocytosis, hemodynamic instability, or temperatures higher than 38°C or lower than 36°C.[53]

The surgical team must be informed about any significant trauma to the driveline, and efforts must be made to effectively immobilize the driveline as soon as possible. Restricting patient activity and a short course of antibiotics may be helpful, although this may predispose to selection of resistant microorganisms. Skin erythema may represent cellulitis even in the absence of seropurulent or purulent drainage. The presence of fever, drainage, progression of erythema, and leukocytosis strongly points to infection as the cause. However, pain and erythema may be produced by inadequate driveline immobilization without infection. Any time this complication is suspected, cultures should be obtained, avoiding deep probing around the driveline track to avoid detaching the host tissues from the driveline surface.

Unfortunately, many times the first indication of the presence of a driveline trauma and infection arrives late, when infection is clinically apparent and a tract is already established around the driveline. Once in this situation, some groups advocate

---

Box 1
Cleveland Clinic classification of ventricular assist device infections

Class I

1. Culture or histologic evidence of infection
   a. Driveline
   b. Pump pocket
   c. Inflow/outflow conduits
2. Bloodstream infection with same organism cultured from the device
3. No other obvious source for the bloodstream infection

Class II

1. Culture or histologic evidence of infection
   a. Driveline
   b. Pump pocket
   c. Inflow/outflow conduits
2. Local or systemic signs of infection
   a. Local: purulent exudates, warmth, erythema, tenderness, induration
   b. Systemic: temperature >38°C, white blood cell count >15,000/mL
3. No bloodstream infection
4. No other obvious source of infection

Class III

1. Local or systemic signs of infection
2. Clinical response to antimicrobials, device removal, or both
3. No culture or histologic evidence of device or bloodstream infection
4. No other obvious source of infection

---

for an aggressive initial surgical management, and report virtually consistent failure of antibiotic treatment together with watchful waiting in this setting.[55] However, regardless of the strategy chosen, intravenous antibiotics should be started as soon as possible to reduce cellulitis before surgical intervention and to reduce the amount of surrounding tissue needing resection.

It is important to ensure that surgical debridement is aggressive enough to avoid leaving behind infected areas that predispose to recurrence, particularly if the device is not going to be completely removed. Planning of the surgical procedure needed in each case may be optimized by preoperative imaging tests. In this setting, a nuclear medicine scan with labeled white cells may help in determining tract anatomy and deciding the amount of tissue that needs to be resected. Indium scanning has also been used similarly in this situation,[56] and computed tomography scanning is also very helpful in identifying occult abscesses and accurately assessing the extension of the infectious process into the abdominal wall and beyond (**Figs. 1** and **2**).

Treatment

When choosing an antibiotic drug regimen, as for other intravascular infections, bactericidal rather than bacteriostatic agents are preferred during the acute phase of treatment. Antibiotic therapy should be guided by culture results, and the narrowest-spectrum drug should be selected once susceptibilities are available to assure longevity of the antibiotic armamentarium and reduce the risk of selection of multidrug-resistant organisms. The authors' protocol for management of driveline infections is described in **Fig. 3**.

The neoepithelialized tissue surrounding the driveline needs to be completely resected, and the tissue excision is extended proximally and circumferentially along the driveline up to a level where complete tissue adherence to the driveline is verified. Sometimes the infected tract extends very deeply, and a complete excision may jeopardize the integrity of the pump pocket. In these

cases an alternative strategy is to perform a partial excision, placing a drain system that leaves a pathway toward the surface to keep the infection draining away from the pump. If the infection extends deeply enough to affect the pump, plans are made based on the patient-specific goal of mechanical support in each case. Pocket infection and abscesses may require drainage of the pump pocket through a new access so that sternotomy healing is not jeopardized, and sometimes LVAD exchange or explant is needed. When long-term antibiotic suppression therapy is used to attempt salvage of the device, it usually requires long courses of parenteral treatment for 6 weeks or longer, depending on response, followed by oral antibiotics for an indefinite period of time.[39] Despite aggressive surgical treatment, repeat revision was needed in 12 of 14 patients in one study, and progressed to pump infection in 6. Permanent healing was achieved in only 3 patients.[3]

Other measures proposed to treat these infections,[57] when complete excision of the infected tract is not possible or when complete healthy tissue apposition around the driveline cannot be accomplished, include frequent dressing changes, establishment of long-term irrigation systems with antimicrobial agents, and relocation of the driveline and exit site in a fresh tunnel. Unfortunately, options available for exit site relocation are limited by the extension of the infection, body habitus, and pump design. This technique has some disadvantages, as it may place deeper segments of the driveline at risk for infection, and may reduce patient mobility or cause discomfort depending on the new location chosen, particularly when moved toward the midline in the abdomen.

Vacuum-assisted closure

A very interesting option that is increasingly being used is vacuum-assisted closure. This method can be used to avoid aggressive surgical treatment in some cases, and as an adjuvant for the previously described techniques. It was first introduced in 1997 by Morykwas and Argenta[58] to treat pressure ulcers and other chronic wounds. The technique applies subatmospheric pressure (−125 mm Hg) on the surface of the wound through a multiperforated drainage tube covered by a sterile polyurethane sponge that adapts to the shape of the defect, and covered with a thin adhesive film that firmly seals the wound from the environment. The dressings are placed on continuous suction and can then undergo uninterrupted treatment for up to 3 days. This situation allows spacing dressing changes, thus reducing wound manipulation and facilitating patient discharge and home therapy.

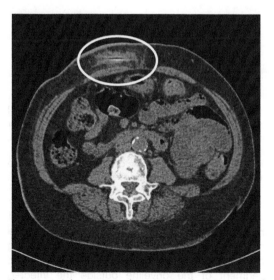

Fig. 1. Axial computed tomography image of a patient with a driveline infection extending from the exit site in the skin into the abdominal subcutaneous tissue. The circled area shows inflammation and stranding of the tissue surrounding the driveline. The inflammatory process extends to the external fascia of the abdominal wall. The muscular layer appears to be preserved.

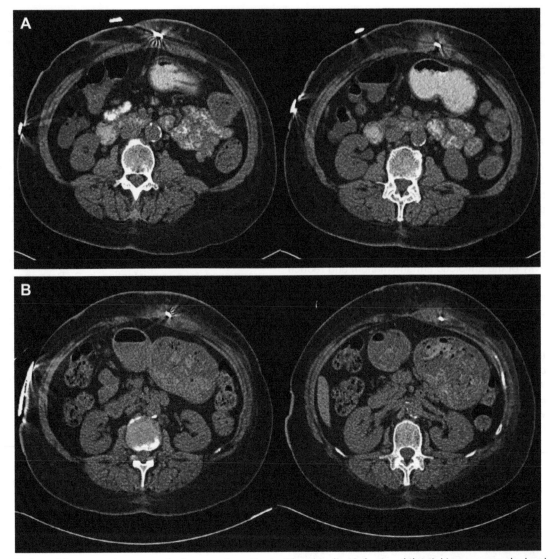

Fig. 2. Axial computed tomography images of a patient with a driveline infection. (*A*) Axial images near the level of the exit site, showing the extension of the inflammatory process through the full extension of the anterior abdominal wall including the rectus sheath. This patient was treated by surgical debridement, exit site relocation, and vacuum-assisted closure. (*B*) After a period of clinical remission, the same patient developed recurrent driveline infection extending into the deeper layers of the abdominal wall with compromise of the pump pocket. The patient was ultimately treated by pump explantation and orthotopic heart transplantation.

The use of subatmospheric pressure to the surface of the wound promotes arteriolar dilatation that stimulates formation of granulation tissue, reduces tissue edema and fluid accumulation, and seals the wound from the exterior to reduce contamination and bacterial colonization. One of the advantages of this system in this particular setting is that it permits one to perform a wide excision of infected tissues with reestablishment of the original driveline tract and exit site. It provides driveline stability and protects the rest of the tract and the pump from external contamination during the granulation and healing process. Other groups prefer to leave the affected segment of the driveline outside the infected tunnel, with its exit site relocated more medially and closer to the pump.[24]

The authors have successfully used this option for treatment of driveline infections and have reported the experience.[57] However, they have observed cases of recurrence of the infection after completion of the vacuum-assisted closure

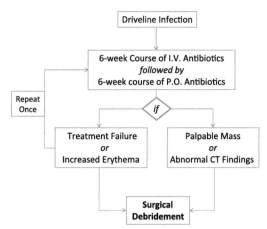

Fig. 3. Algorithm for the management of driveline infections. CT, computed tomography; I.V., intravenous; P.O., by mouth.

therapy and closure of the skin over the driveline (see **Fig. 2**).

The authors have recently reviewed their institutional experience on this subject. From June 2000 to May 2009, a total of 133 LVADs were implanted. Continuous-flow LVADs were used in 86 patients (65%) and 47 patients (35%) received a pulsatile-flow device. Driveline infection was diagnosed in 43 patients (32%) and 22 patients required surgical debridement. Among those patients who underwent debridement, repeated surgical debridement was required in 12 patients. Freedom from driveline infection in the series was 33% at 18-month follow-up.

In the subgroup of patients receiving a continuous-flow LVAD, driveline infection was diagnosed in 26 patients (30%) and debridement was required in 17 patients (20%). Repeated debridement procedures were required in 10 patients in this cohort, highlighting the insidious nature of this complication. Among patients implanted with a continuous-flow LVAD, none of the cases of driveline infection appeared before 30 days after the implant. Furthermore, driveline infection appeared after more than 90 days from the implant in 24 of the total of 26 patients who had this complication.

SUMMARY

Driveline infections have emerged as the most important infectious complication of mechanical circulatory support in the modern era. Despite advances in device technology and treatment, infection continues to have important implications negatively influencing survival, quality of life, patient autonomy, and monetary cost. Driveline infection

may ultimately endanger the final objective of mechanical assist device therapy.

Prevention is the most efficient measure to fight against driveline infection after LVAD implantation. Prevention must start even before the surgical implant, with measures directed to improve the patient's underlying condition and avoid colonization with microorganisms. Postoperative efforts must be centered on driveline immobilization to promote healing of the host tissues and integration around the driveline surface.

Early recognition of driveline infection and prompt treatment are key to the success of all therapeutic measures, including surgical debridement. Surgery, when needed, has to provide adequate removal of infected material as well as appropriate conditions for healing of the new driveline path and exit site.

REFERENCES

1. Rose EA, Gelijns AC, Moskowitz AJ, et al. Long-term use of a left ventricular assist device for end-stage heart failure. N Engl J Med 2001;345(20):1435–43.
2. DeRose JJ, Argenziano M, Sun BC, et al. Implantable left ventricular assist devices: an evolving long-term cardiac replacement therapy. Ann Surg 1997;226(4):461–8 [discussion: 468–70].
3. Zierer A, Melby SJ, Voeller RK, et al. Late-onset driveline infections: the Achilles' heel of prolonged left ventricular assist device support. Ann Thorac Surg 2007;84(2):515–20.
4. Gordon SM, Schmitt SK, Jacobs M, et al. Nosocomial bloodstream infections in patients with implantable left ventricular assist devices. Ann Thorac Surg 2001;72(3):725–30.
5. Oz MC, Gelijns AC, Miller L, et al. Left ventricular assist devices as permanent heart failure therapy: the price of progress. Ann Surg 2003;238(4):577–83 [discussion: 583–5].
6. Elek SD, Conen PE. The virulence of *Staphylococcus pyogenes* for man; a study of the problems of wound infection. Br J Exp Pathol 1957;38(6):573–86.
7. Didisheim P. Current concepts of thrombosis and infection in artificial organs. ASAIO J 1994;40(2):230–7.
8. Interagency Registry for Mechanically Assisted Circulatory Support (INTERMACS). Manual of operations version 2.3. Appendix A: Adverse event definitions. Available at: http://www.intermacs.org/2008. 5. Accessed August 1, 2011.
9. John R, Pagani FD, Naka Y, et al. Post-cardiac transplant survival after support with a continuous-flow left ventricular assist device: impact of duration of left ventricular assist device support and other variables. J Thorac Cardiovasc Surg 2010;140(1):174–81.
10. McCarthy PM, Schmitt SK, Vargo RL, et al. Implantable LVAD infections: implications for permanent use of the

device. Ann Thorac Surg 1996;61(1):359–65 [discussion: 372–3].

11. Griffith BP, Kormos RL, Nastala CJ, et al. Results of extended bridge to transplantation: window into the future of permanent ventricular assist devices. Ann Thorac Surg 1996;61(1):396–8 [discussion: 407].

12. Oaks TE, Pae WE Jr, Miller CA, et al. Combined registry for the clinical use of mechanical ventricular assist pumps and the total artificial heart in conjunction with heart transplantation: fifth official report—1990. J Heart Lung Transplant 1991;10(5 Pt 1):621–5.

13. Argenziano M, Catanese KA, Moazami N, et al. The influence of infection on survival and successful transplantation in patients with left ventricular assist devices. J Heart Lung Transplant 1997;16(8):822–31.

14. Prendergast TW, Todd BA, Beyer AJ 3rd, et al. Management of left ventricular assist device infection with heart transplantation. Ann Thorac Surg 1997;64(1):142–7.

15. Chinn R, Dembitsky W, Eaton L, et al. Multicenter experience: prevention and management of left ventricular assist device infections. ASAIO J 2005;51(4):461–70.

16. Holman WL, Park SJ, Long JW, et al. Infection in permanent circulatory support: experience from the REMATCH trial. J Heart Lung Transplant 2004;23(12):1359–65.

17. Miller LW, Pagani FD, Russell SD, et al. Use of a continuous-flow device in patients awaiting heart transplantation. N Engl J Med 2007;357(9):885–96.

18. Raymond AL, Kfoury AG, Bishop CJ, et al. Obesity and left ventricular assist device driveline exit site infection. ASAIO J 2010;56(1):57–60.

19. Gordon RJ, Quagliarello B, Lowy FD. Ventricular assist device-related infections. Lancet Infect Dis 2006;6(7):426–37.

20. Simon D, Fischer S, Grossman A, et al. Left ventricular assist device-related infection: treatment and outcome. Clin Infect Dis 2005;40(8):1108–15.

21. Jarvik R, Westaby S, Katsumata T, et al. LVAD power delivery: a percutaneous approach to avoid infection. Ann Thorac Surg 1998;65(2):470–3.

22. Gristina AG, Giridhar G, Gabriel BL, et al. Cell biology and molecular mechanisms in artificial device infections. Int J Artif Organs 1993;16(11):755–63.

23. Choi L, Choudhri AF, Pillarisetty VG, et al. Development of an infection-resistant LVAD driveline: a novel approach to the prevention of device-related infections. J Heart Lung Transplant 1999;18(11):1103–10.

24. Garatti A, Giuseppe B, Russo CF, et al. Drive-line exit-site infection in a patient with axial-flow pump support: successful management using vacuum-assisted therapy. J Heart Lung Transplant 2007;26(9):956–9.

25. Sun BC, Catanese KA, Spanier TB, et al. 100 long-term implantable left ventricular assist devices: the Columbia Presbyterian interim experience. Ann Thorac Surg 1999;68(2):688–94.

26. Hetzer R, Weng Y, Potapov EV, et al. First experiences with a novel magnetically suspended axial flow left ventricular assist device. Eur J Cardiothorac Surg 2004;25(6):964–70.

27. Siegenthaler MP, Martin J, Pernice K, et al. The Jarvik 2000 is associated with less infections than the HeartMate left ventricular assist device. Eur J Cardiothorac Surg 2003;23(5):748–54 [discussion: 754–5].

28. Vitali E, Lanfranconi M, Ribera E, et al. Successful experience in bridging patients to heart transplantation with the MicroMed DeBakey ventricular assist device. Ann Thorac Surg 2003;75(4):1200–4.

29. Maki DG, Stolz SM, Wheeler S, et al. Prevention of central venous catheter-related bloodstream infection by use of an antiseptic-impregnated catheter. A randomized, controlled trial. Ann Intern Med 1997;127(4):257–66.

30. McKellar SH, Allred BD, Marks JD, et al. Treatment of infected left ventricular assist device using antibiotic-impregnated beads. Ann Thorac Surg 1999;67(2):554–5.

31. Westaby S, Siegenthaler M, Beyersdorf F, et al. Destination therapy with a rotary blood pump and novel power delivery. Eur J Cardiothorac Surg 2010;37(2):350–6.

32. Gesler W, Smith R, DeDecker PG, et al. Updated feasibility trial experience with the Viaderm percutaneous access device. ASAIO J 2004;50(4):349–53.

33. Okamoto E, Yamamoto Y, Akasaka Y, et al. A new transcutaneous energy transmission system with hybrid energy coils for driving an implantable biventricular assist device. Artif Organs 2009;33(8):622–6.

34. Rintoul TC, Dolgin A. Thoratec transcutaneous energy transformer system: a review and update. ASAIO J 2004;50(4):397–400.

35. Slaughter MS, Myers TJ. Transcutaneous energy transmission for mechanical circulatory support systems: history, current status, and future prospects. J Card Surg 2010;25(4):484–9.

36. Patti JM, Allen BL, McGavin MJ, et al. MSCRAMM-mediated adherence of microorganisms to host tissues. Annu Rev Microbiol 1994;48:585–617.

37. Padera RF. Infection in ventricular assist devices: the role of biofilm. Cardiovasc Pathol 2006;15(5):264–70.

38. Arrecubieta C, Toba FA, von Bayern M, et al. SdrF, a *Staphylococcus epidermidis* surface protein, contributes to the initiation of ventricular assist device driveline-related infections. PLoS Pathog 2009;5(5):e1000411.

39. Shoham S, Miller LW. Cardiac assist device infections. Curr Infect Dis Rep 2009;11(4):268–73.

40. Costerton JW, Lewandowski Z, Caldwell DE, et al. Microbial biofilms. Annu Rev Microbiol 1995;49:711–45.

41. Dasgupta MK. Biofilms and infection in dialysis patients. Semin Dial 2002;15(5):338–46.

42. Hall-Stoodley L, Costerton JW, Stoodley P. Bacterial biofilms: from the natural environment to infectious diseases. Nat Rev Microbiol 2004;2(2):95–108.

43. Otto M. Staphylococcus epidermidis—the 'accidental' pathogen. Nat Rev Microbiol 2009;7(8):555–67.

44. Toba FA, Akashi H, Arrecubieta C, et al. Role of biofilm in Staphylococcus aureus and Staphylococcus epidermidis ventricular assist device driveline infections. J Thorac Cardiovasc Surg 2011;141(5):1259–64.

45. Dickinson GM, Bisno AL. Infections associated with prosthetic devices: clinical considerations. Int J Artif Organs 1993;16(11):749–54.

46. Richards GK, Gagnon RF. An assay of Staphylococcus epidermidis biofilm responses to therapeutic agents. Int J Artif Organs 1993;16(11):777–88.

47. Costerton JW, Khoury AE, Ward KH, et al. Practical measures to control device-related bacterial infections. Int J Artif Organs 1993;16(11):765–70.

48. Ankersmit HJ, Edwards NM, Schuster M, et al. Quantitative changes in T-cell populations after left ventricular assist device implantation: relationship to T-cell apoptosis and soluble CD95. Circulation 1999;100(19 Suppl):II211–5.

49. Ankersmit HJ, Tugulea S, Spanier T, et al. Activation-induced T-cell death and immune dysfunction after implantation of left-ventricular assist device. Lancet 1999;354(9178):550–5.

50. Kimball PM, Flattery M, McDougan F, et al. Cellular immunity impaired among patients on left ventricular assist device for 6 months. Ann Thorac Surg 2008; 85(5):1656–61.

51. Yamani MH, Chuang HH, Ozduran V, et al. The impact of hypogammaglobulinemia on infection outcome in patients undergoing ventricular assist device implantation. J Heart Lung Transplant 2006; 25(7):820–4.

52. Bratzler DW, Houck PM. Antimicrobial prophylaxis for surgery: an advisory statement from the National Surgical Infection Prevention Project. Clin Infect Dis 2004;38(12):1706–15.

53. Schaffer JM, Allen JG, Weiss ES, et al. Infectious complications after pulsatile-flow and continuous-flow left ventricular assist device implantation. J Heart Lung Transplant 2011;30(2):164–74.

54. Tjan TD, Asfour B, Hammel D, et al. Wound complications after left ventricular assist device implantation. Ann Thorac Surg 2000;70(2):538–41.

55. Pasque MK, Hanselman T, Shelton K, et al. Surgical management of Novacor drive-line exit site infections. Ann Thorac Surg 2002;74(4):1267–8.

56. Baradarian S, Stahovich M, Krause S, et al. Case series: clinical management of persistent mechanical assist device driveline drainage using vacuum-assisted closure therapy. ASAIO J 2006;52(3):354–6.

57. Yuh DD, Albaugh M, Ullrich S, et al. Treatment of ventricular assist device driveline infection with vacuum-assisted closure system. Ann Thorac Surg 2005;80(4):1493–5.

58. Argenta LC, Morykwas MJ. Vacuum-assisted closure: a new method for wound control and treatment: clinical experience. Ann Plast Surg 1997; 38(6):563–76 [discussion: 577].

59. Martin SI, Wellington L, Stevenson KB, et al. Effect of body mass index and device type on infection in left ventricular assist device support beyond 30 days. Interact Cardiovasc Thorac Surg 2010;11(1):20–3.

60. Holman WL, Kirklin JK, Naftel DC, et al. Infection after implantation of pulsatile mechanical circulatory support devices. J Thorac Cardiovasc Surg 2010; 139(6):1632–1636.e2.

61. Aslam S, Hernandez M, Thornby J, et al. Risk factors and outcomes of fungal ventricular-assist device infections. Clin Infect Dis 2010;50(5):664–71.

62. Saito S, Matsumiya G, Sakaguchi T, et al. Risk factor analysis of long-term support with left ventricular assist system. Circ J 2010;74(4):715–22.

63. Pagani FD, Miller LW, Russell SD, et al. Extended mechanical circulatory support with a continuous-flow rotary left ventricular assist device. J Am Coll Cardiol 2009;54(4):312–21.

64. Morshuis M, El-Banayosy A, Arusoglu L, et al. European experience of DuraHeart magnetically levitated centrifugal left ventricular assist system. Eur J Cardiothorac Surg 2009;35(6):1020–7 [discussion: 1027–8].

65. Pae WE, Connell JM, Adelowo A, et al. Does total implantability reduce infection with the use of a left ventricular assist device? The LionHeart experience in Europe. J Heart Lung Transplant 2007; 26(3):219–29.

66. Monkowski DH, Axelrod P, Fekete T, et al. Infections associated with ventricular assist devices: epidemiology and effect on prognosis after transplantation. Transpl Infect Dis 2007;9(2):114–20.

Editorial Comments on "Left-Ventricular Assist Device Driveline Infections"

John A. Elefteriades, MD

KEY CONCEPTS

Drs Daniel Pereda and John V. Conte, the authors of "Left-Ventricular Assist Device Driveline Infections," outline clearly and in detail the pathogenesis, etiology, microbiology, recognition, and treatment of driveline infections. The investigators clarify how prevalent these infections are and how strong an impact they have on survival and effective transition to transplantation. The authors outline important concepts, including

- Prevention (preoperative optimization by surveillance cultures, nutrition, and prophylactic antibiotics; small skin opening, with tight purse-string sutures; and postoperative aseptic technique and driveline immobilization)
- Recognition (poor tissue adherence, erythema, drainage, abnormalities on computed tomographic scan)
- Treatment (from enhanced local care to antibiotics to surgical debridement of the driveline or LVAD removal or accelerated transplantation).

STRENGTHS

This article is an encyclopedic and insightful review of this important topic.

WEAKNESSES

There is no strong evidence that any prophylactic or therapeutic measures are clearly and conclusively effective.

Section of Cardiac Surgery, Yale University School of Medicine, Boardman 2, 333 Cedar Street, New Haven, CT 06510, USA
E-mail address: john.elefteriades@yale.edu

Cardiol Clin 29 (2011) 529
doi:10.1016/j.ccl.2011.07.004
0733-8651/11/$ – see front matter © 2011 Published by Elsevier Inc.

Bridge to Recovery: What Remains to be Discovered?

Michael Ibrahim, BA (Cantab),
Cesare M. Terracciano, MD, PhD, Magdi H. Yacoub, FRS*

KEYWORDS

- LVAD • Cardiac recovery • Mechanical unloading
- Harefield protocol

Progress in science and medicine is often marked by imaginative leaps, followed by a process of slow, possibly painful, validation. Bridge to recovery (BTR) is a prime example of such processes. Following the original observation that some patients can develop "myocardial recovery" during left ventricular assist device (LVAD) support alone or in combination with other forms of therapy, an extensive effort to establish this potentially extremely valuable method of treating advanced heart failure ensued. This consisted of concerted efforts to define the extensive structural, molecular, and biochemical changes during unloading (ie, reverse remodeling); as well as the timing, influence on functional changes, clinical features, and putative mechanisms. This resulted in the accumulation of a wealth of knowledge with implications beyond establishing BTR. This knowledge offers unprecedented opportunities to discover the basic mechanisms of heart failure, its progression, and regression. This article attempts to review what has been learned during this incredibly productive period and what remains to be discovered.

HISTORICAL PERSPECTIVE

Heart failure continues to be one of the major causes of death and disability worldwide.[1] In its advanced stage, heart failure carries an extremely poor prognosis with the only effective treatment being cardiac transplantation. Unfortunately, this form of treatment is hampered by the scarcity and unpredictable availability of donor organs.

This stimulated the development of LVADs as a bridge or alternative to transplantation. In this setting, the seminal discovery of BTR was accidentally made.[2,3] At this point, the rates of recovery seem to be low.[4–6] However, these rates are substantially increased by combining LVAD treatment with pharmacologic therapy.[7,8] In spite of these exciting discoveries, the procedure remains underused, with many unanswered questions. These questions include the following: which patients, which device, under what mode of operation, and unloaded for how long? Additionally, this mode of therapy requires developing tests for myocardial recovery, developing methods of device explantation, and understanding long-term outcomes and possible mechanisms of recovery. Answering these questions is critical to progress in the field, and beyond.

Application and Resource Allocation

Success in this field requires the services of a dedicated team experienced in the management of advanced heart failure, including LVADs and cardiac transplantation, who can stimulate and closely monitor the process of recovery. In addition, the involvement of basic science research laboratories is essential.[9] Unfortunately, one or more of these components is frequently absent. In addition, the attraction of performing transplantation, which is perceived to be a more established procedure, has hampered the wider application of BTR. On the other hand, the fact that, following

The authors have nothing to disclose.
Heart Science Centre, Magdi Yacoub Institute, Harefield Hospital, Hill End Road, LONDON UB9 6JH, UK
* Corresponding author.
E-mail address: m.yacoub@imperial.ac.uk

Cardiol Clin 29 (2011) 531–547
doi:10.1016/j.ccl.2011.08.007
0733-8651/11/$ – see front matter © 2011 Elsevier Inc. All rights reserved

BTR, patients retain their native innervated heart and do not receive immunosuppressive drugs or high levels of anticoagulation are regarded as great advantages.

CURRENT INDICATIONS
For Whom?

The indications for BTR are still evolving. To date, BTR has been offered mainly to patients with severe heart failure due to nonischemic dilated cardiomyopathy (DCM); whether idiopathic, postviral, familial, postpartum, or after chemotherapy; and regardless of age, sex, or duration of heart failure. In approximately 40% of patients with idiopathic DCM, the origin is familial, with or without defined genetic mutations.[10] Patients with heart failure following chemotherapy, who were previously thought to have irreversible myocardial damage,[11] have proved to be good candidates for BTR. Postpartum cardiomyopathy represents a wide spectrum of disease,[12] with some responding to medical therapy and others requiring LVAD therapy. In that subset of patients, recovery has been observed.[8] Patients with active myocarditis are usually excluded because they usually recover spontaneously following intensive medical therapy. Out of the large pool of patients with ischemic cardiomyopathy, a significant minority who have single-vessel disease or previously revascularized viable myocardium in the absence of extensive fibrosis and scarring could be candidates for BTR.[13,14]

Timing?

One of the most important issues in the clinical use of LVADs is the decision about the timing of application of this potentially powerful form of therapy. Some practitioners advocate increased use of LVADs in healthier patients[15] and other practitioners await more clinical evidence supporting LVAD therapy in less severe heart failure.[16] Timing of LVAD intervention can have an important influence on outcome, in the short-term and the long-term. In an attempt to guide decision-making, several prognostic indicators and clinical classifications of advanced heart failure, such as the Interagency Registry for Mechanically Assisted Circulatory Support (INTERMACS) grading system (**Table 1**),[17] have been introduced. Virtually all patients recruited for BTR are from the larger pool of bridge-to-transplantation patients, and, by definition, have an extremely advanced grade of heart failure (INTERMACS profile 1–3). This high severity can have an adverse effect on early mortality, which is usually caused by multiorgan damage. Operating on patients at an earlier stage

of the disease is currently being hotly debated[15,16] and depends on balancing the moving target of device-related complications with the expected benefits of early operation.

Which Device?

Rapid progress in the field has resulted in the development of several types of implantable LVADs (**Fig. 1**) with different performance characteristics that can influence the mode and degree of interaction with the native heart.[18] The currently available devices include three types (generations): pulsatile, impeller, and centrifugal pumps. Although the pulsatile devices such as Heart Mate I are thought to provide better unloading of the left ventricle (LV), which could enhance recovery, their use has declined owing to their much bigger size and higher incidence of mechanical complications.[18] Recent series using the continuous-flow Heart Mate II reported results similar to those obtained by Heart Mate I.[19] Further definition of the hemodynamic interaction between the device and the native heart (**Figs. 2** and **3**) should help in optimizing the choice of device.

MODE OF OPERATION

Although some of the pulsatile devices can be synchronized with the native heart to provide counter pulsation, this facility is hardly ever used. In these patients, the aortic valve remains closed most of the time, with occasional ejection from the LV. Device ejection involves closure of the device inflow valve, which allows filling of the LV and, therefore, ventricular ejection (see **Figs. 2** and **3**). It is important not to allow the systemic pressure to rise, which could damage the already diseased LV. With continuous-flow pumps, the speed of the device should be adjusted to allow adequate flow and unloading without allowing the ventricle to be sucked flat, which can cause ventricular arrhythmia and damage to the ventricular wall. The patient should be encouraged to undergo regular exercise using a formal rehabilitation program. This should help to condition skeletal muscle and possibly induce physiologic cardiac hypertrophy. The value of gradually reloading the heart by gradually reducing the speed of the pump has not been tested.

How Long to Monitor Recovery?

Although the process of reverse remodelling starts within a very short time after instituting unloading, it continues for many weeks or months and varies in different types of animal models and in patterns observed in humans,[5,20] with relatively

Table 1
INTERMACS: profiles for patient selection

Profile	Description	Possible Profile Modifiers		
		Temporary Circulatory Support (TCS)	Arrhythmia (A)	Frequent Flyer (FF)
—	—			
1.	Critical cardiogenic shock	X	X	—
2.	Progressive decline on inotropic support	X	X	—
3.	Stable but inotrope dependent	X (in hospital)	X	X (if home)
4.	Resting symptoms, home on oral therapy	—	X	X
5.	Exertion intolerant	—	X	X
6.	Exertion limited	—	X	X
7.	Advanced New York Heart Association class III symptoms	—	X	—

INTERMACS provides a convenient, clinically relevant structure for describing patients who are not responding to optimal heart failure medication and may be candidates for LVAD support. Patients are described in seven categories and there are three modifiers for the more severe groups: temporary circulatory support (TCS), the presence of arrhythmia (A), and frequent rehospitalization (FF).
   Data from Stevenson LW, Pagani FD, Young JB et al. INTERMACS profiles of advanced heart failure: the current picture. J Heart Lung Transplant 2009;28:535–41.

wide variations between individuals. This highlights the importance of monitoring recovery using accurate methods for adequate periods of time. Several methods for testing recovery have been developed that depend on the type of device and the state of the patient. The tests are usually started 4 weeks after leaving intensive care, when the patient is fully ambulant with no evidence of infection or any other complication. Measuring LV size and ejection fraction (LVEF) during LVAD support provides a rough estimate of the degree of recovery.[21] However, accurate evaluation of cardiac function requires discontinuing the contribution to cardiac output by the device. This can be achieved by switching the device off in pulsatile pumps or by reducing the revolutions per minute in continuous-flow pumps. This should be performed after full heparinization, with close monitoring of hemodynamic and ECG parameters.[22] If the patient tolerates this period, a 6-minute walk test is followed by another ECG to test for inotropic reserve. These tests are repeated at biweekly intervals and continued for up to 18 months so long as there is any degree of improvement in the parameters measured. Additional tests measuring exercise capacity with gas exchange and cardiac catheterization are performed at the appropriate stages to confirm recovery.[8]

COMBINATION THERAPY: THE HAREFIELD PROTOCOL

One limitation of prolonged mechanical unloading is thought to be cardiac atrophy,[23] which implies

functional deterioration associated with reductions in organ and cardiomyocyte size. We showed that prolonged mechanical unloading in an animal model results in atrophic remodeling and blunted contractility[24] due to pathologic remodeling of cellular Ca^{2+} handling.[25] It was hypothesized that the beta-2 adrenergic agonist, clenbuterol could prevent unloading-induced atrophy. A two-stage process was devised that aimed at, first, inducing maximal reverse remodeling and, second, preventing atrophy using clenbuterol. This strategy achieved a 75% recovery rate in a selected patient cohort of 15 non-ischemic patients.[8,19] Since this clinical study, the cellular and molecular effects of clenbuterol in experimental studies has been examined. It was found that clenbuterol augmented the Ca^{2+} transient amplitude, promoted the expression of a number of Ca^{2+} handling proteins (including Sarcoplasmic reticulum Ca^{2+} ATPase 2a [SERCA 2a] and Sodium-Calcium Exchanger [NCX]), and increased sarcoplasmic reticular stores of Ca^{2+}.[26] Clenbuterol also enhanced myofilament sensitivity to Ca^{2+} in the setting of heart failure.[27] Clenbuterol may also promote physiologic hypertrophy via increased insulin-like growth factor-1 (IGF-1) levels.[28]

Criteria for Explantation and Durability of Recovery After LVAD Explantation

Specific criteria based on ECG, cardiac catheterization, and other assessments guide the explantation criteria and description of recovery. At the Harefield Hospital, the specific criteria used is

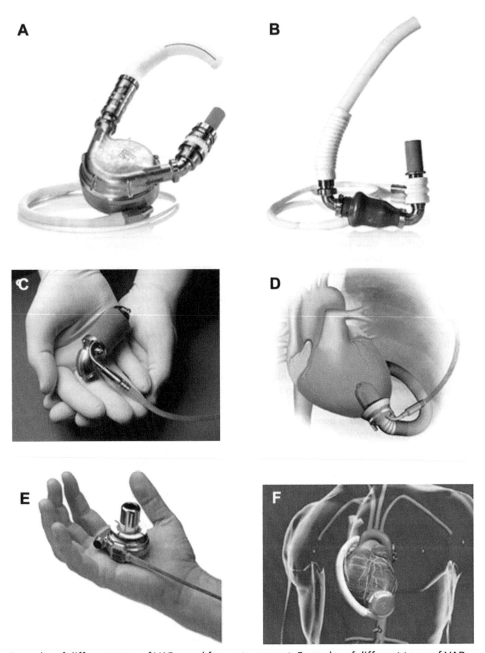

Fig. 1. Examples of different types of VADs used for acute support. Examples of different types of VADs used for longer-term support. (*A, B*) Examples of first-generation pulsatile (HeartMate I or XVE, Thoratec Corp) and second-generation continuous-flow (HeartMate II, Thoratec Corp, CA, USA). VADs used with abdominal implantation (from http://www.thoratec.com). (*C, D*) A second-generation LVAD (Jarvik 2000, Jarvik Heart [Jarvik, NY, USA]) with intraventricular implantation (http://www.jarvikheart.com). (*E, F*) A third-generation centrifugal VAD (HVAD, HeartWare, MA, USA, http://www.heartware.com.au), with small dimension and hydrodynamically suspended impeller. (*From* Terracciano CM, Miller LW, Yacoub MH. Contemporary use of ventricular assist devices. Annu Rev Med 2010;61:255–70; with permission.)

LVEF greater than 45%, LVEDd less than 60 mm, LV end-systolic diameter less than 50 mm, pulmonary capillary wedge pressure less than 12 mm Hg, cardiac index greater than 2.8 l min-1, and a VO$_2$ max of greater than 16 mL kg-1 min-1 during off-pump testing to be predictive of stable recovery.[19] Dobutamine stress testing for the assessment of cardiac recovery

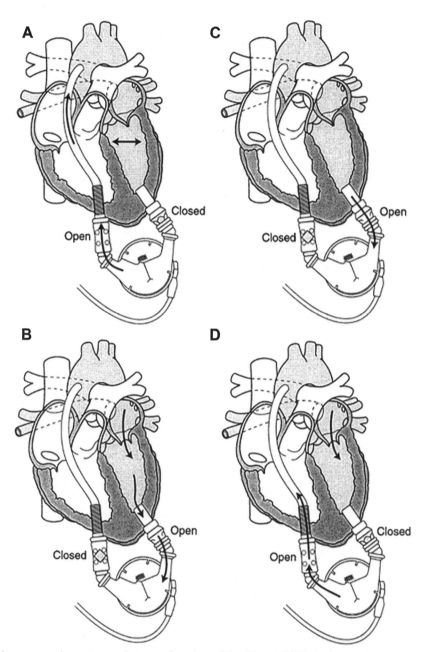

Fig. 2. Synchronous and counter-synchronous function of the LV and LVAD. In the synchronous state, when LV systole coincides with device ejection, systole closes the mitral valve but fails to open the aortic valve. Because the inlet valve of the device is closed, LV contraction is isovolumic and wall motion, which must reflect incoordinate contraction, is reduced. (A) Device and LV filling occur simultaneously, resulting in continuous flow through the mitral valve during diastole. (B) In the counter-synchronous state, during LV systole the ventricle contracts, closing the mitral valve, and it ejects blood into the LVAD via the inlet valve, thus augmenting filling of the device. (C) LV wall motion is maximal. LV filling occurs during device ejection and the device inlet valve is closed so that LV pressure rises normally and the mitral flow pattern is normal. (D) If the LV were to generate sufficient pressure to open the native aortic valve, parallel ejection could occur from the both the LV and the LVAD.

has also been successfully utilized at the Texas Heart Institute.[29] The ultimate test of cardiac recovery is freedom from heart failure after device explantation.

There are currently no specific biologic markers of recovery. Assessment is based on clinical parameters alone. Therefore, the assessment of the durability of relief from heart failure is based on

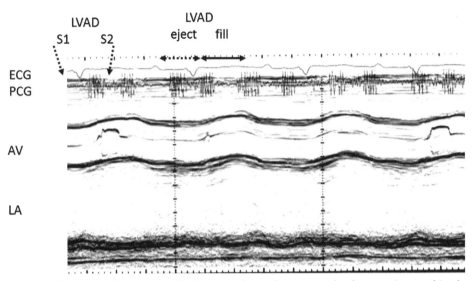

Fig. 3. An M-mode ECG showing relationship between hemodynamics and valve opening. In this plane, it is possible to observe the timing of ventricular electrical activity, the opening of the aortic valve, and the phonocardiogram (PCG) recording. AV, aortic valve; LA, left atrium.

regular clinical assessment. Identifying patients who are likely to relapse to heart failure (thus, assessing the probable durability of relief from heart failure) is an important issue. Clarification is likely to give greater confidence to patients and physicians considering device explantation. One study, which followed patients up to 15 years after device explantation, showed that recurrence of heart failure was more likely when duration of LVAD therapy exceeded 25 months and when latest pre-explantation ECG assessment showed an impaired and dilated ventricle (LVEF<45% and LV end-diastolic diameter [LVEDd]>55 mm).[30] Other predictors of poor durability of recovery were a greater than 10% decrease in relative wall thickness (RWT) (ie, interventricular septum thickness plus posterior wall thickness, or LVEDd), RWT less than 0.38, and heart failure duration of greater than 5 years. In a recent study from Harefield Hospital, we obtained an estimated 83.3% freedom from heart failure 3 years postexplantation.[19] There is evidence that a rapid recovery is more durable after explantation.[31]

Little is known of the quality of life of patients who have recovered from heart failure after LVAD therapy. LVAD therapy used as a destination therapy had been shown to improve quality of life in patients with New York Heart Association class IV heart failure.[32] Whether quality of life is better, worse, or the same for patients who had been on LVAD support and have been subsequently explanted as BTR is not well studied.

The Biologic Mechanisms of Cardiac Recovery

Since the phenomenon of cardiac recovery was discovered at the clinical level, efforts in the laboratory have attempted to define its mechanisms. Patients treated with LVADs offer the unprecedented opportunity to study myocardial structure and biology at two time points in the same patient: before treatment (tissue taken during device implantation) and after treatment (tissue taken at explantation or transplantation). Given the limited amount of tissue available at explantation in BTR patients, most of the studies have been performed on bridge-to-transplantation samples and it is, therefore, difficult to correlate the relationship between the changes observed and clinical consequences. Improvements in the ability to assess myocardial performance in VAD-treated patients clinically and the opportunity to study myocardial samples from the same patients are crucial to determine the exact series of events that leads to favorable myocardial remodeling and clinical recovery.

Reverse remodeling is associated with changes in the myocardium at multiple levels: whole organ, tissue, cellular, and molecular. Some of these changes play major mechanistic roles in reverse remodeling, whereas others are epiphenomena. To clarify this issue, observational studies in humans should be supplemented by laboratory studies involving animal models and in vitro experiments. The "main players" in the process of reverse remodeling include the cardiomyocytes, the extracellular matrix (ECM), the fibroblasts, and the microvascular system, as well as neuroendocrine mechanisms.

Cardiomyocyte Structure and Function

Because the cardiomyocytes contain the contractile machinery, they have been extensively studied in terms of their size, shape, and function. Several methods of measuring cell size are in use, including using intact tissue sections[7] or isolated cells,[33] or applying standard morphometric or electrophysiological techniques[34] (such as measuring cell capacitance during patch-clamping). Regression of both cardiac (**Fig. 4**) and cardiomyocyte hypertrophy has been documented after LVAD therapy.[35,36] In heart failure, hypertrophy at organ and cellular levels is associated with poor prognosis. It is widely assumed that regression in hypertrophy improves prognosis, partly because of LVAD studies that show both regression of cellular hypertrophy and improvements in functional features such as cellular contractility,[33] which can be measured in several ways. However, in a study where we compared cellular features in patients who, after LVAD therapy and the Harefield Protocol, had recovered clinically and those who did not, we did not find that regression of cellular hypertrophy was associated with clinical recovery.[34] Instead, regression of cellular hypertrophy occurred in both groups. Determinants of recovery included the sarcoplasmic reticulum Ca^{2+} content, a major determinant of cellular contractility,[34] which is depressed in heart failure.[37] Reuptake of diastolic Ca^{2+} into the sarcoplasmic reticulum (SR) is mediated by sarcoplasmic endoreticulum Ca^{2+} ATPase 2a (SERCA 2a) and is impaired in heart failure and is improved after LVAD therapy (**Fig. 5**).[2,33]

Cell shape may also play a role in reverse remodeling induced by mechanical unloading. Recently, it was reported that reverse remodeling of specialized structures in the cell membrane (the transverse tubules, which are required for excitation-contraction coupling and are damaged in human heart failure,[38] as well as cellular Ca^{2+} handling) occurs after mechanical unloading of heart failure in a rodent model (**Fig. 6**).[39] Whether these changes occur and are relevant in the clinical improvements observed after LVAD therapy is not known.

Innate Immune System

The innate immune system is an evolutionarily old system of multiple genetically predetermined receptors that recognize specific highly preserved sequences termed pathogen-associated molecular patterns (PAMPS). The innate immune system receptors (eg, toll-like receptor 4 [TLR4]) that recognize these patterns activate several molecules with wide-ranging effects, including on the myocardium. TLR4; tumor necrosis factor α (TNFα); and interleukins (IL)-6 and IL-1β have all shown cardio-depressive effects. In search of molecular markers for cardiac decompensation requiring LVAD insertion, the expression of TL4, TNFα, IL6, and IL-1β in stable patients compared with those requiring LVAD insertion was investigated.[40] It was found that there was a relative increase in these molecules in patients requiring LVAD insertion compared with those with stable heart failure, suggesting that activation of the innate immune system occurs in these patients (**Fig. 7**). Assessment of these (and other[41]) markers may allow more refined, and earlier, selection of patients for LVAD therapy, which

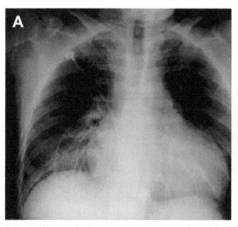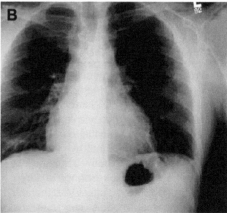

Fig. 4. Chest radiograph showing regression of cardiac dilatation after LVAD support. (*A*) Pre-LVAD implantation. (*B*) Post-LVAD support. (*From* Razeghi P, Myers TJ, Frazier OH, et al. Reverse remodeling of the failing human heart with mechanical unloading. Cardiology 2002;98:167–74; with permission.)

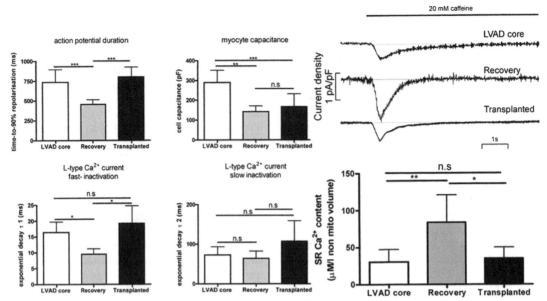

Fig. 5. Clinical recovery correlates with Ca^{2+} handling changes, not regression of cellular hypertrophy Main panel: electrophysiological parameters of myocytes isolated from LVAD cores and tissue from explanted (recovery) and transplanted hearts without recovery. Top right, cell capacitance; left, AP duration; bottom, fast (*left*) and slow (*right*) components of inactivation of Ca^{2+} current. * $P<.05$; ** $P<.01$; *** $P<.001$. Right panel: SR Ca^{2+} content from myocytes isolated from LVAD cores and tissue from explanted (recovery) and transplanted hearts without recovery. Cells were voltage-clamped at their resting membrane potentials. A train stimulation protocol (30 voltage clamp steps from –80 to 0 mV [500 ms] at 1 Hz) preceded rapid application of 20 mmol/L caffeine. Bottom, mean values±SD of calculated SR Ca^{2+} content. * $P<.05$; ** $P<.01$. (*From* Terracciano CM, Hardy J, Birks EJ, Khaghani A, Banner NR, Yacoub MH. Clinical recovery from end-stage heart failure using left-ventricular assist device and pharmacologic therapy correlates with increased sarcoplasmic reticulum calcium content but not with regression of cellular hypertrophy. Circulation 2004;109:2263–5; with permission.)

could enhance the chances of myocardial recovery. Modulating cytokine production or activation of the innate immune response by blocking TLR4 activation may prevent disease progression. This could be used in conjunction with LVAD therapy to enhance recovery. There is some evidence that LVADs may suppress proinflammatory cytokine responses in animal models of heart failure.[42]

Myocardial Electrophysiology and Cellular Excitation-Contraction Coupling

Reverse electrophysiological remodelling occurs at the myocardial level during LVAD therapy as demonstrated by the reduction of the QT interval. Reverse remodelling also occurs at myocyte level as evidenced by reduced action potential duration and by improved L-type Ca^{2+} channel dynamics.[43,44] Several studies report that both basal cellular contractility and the contractile response to adrenergic stimulation[33] are improved after LVAD therapy. Recent work in animal models suggests that the transverse tubule system, which is essential in mediating the close relationship between the L-type Ca^{2+} channels and Ryanodine receptors, is

sensitive to mechanical load and may undergo reverse remodeling during mechanical unloading.[25,39,45] Whether this also true in humans is not known. Further work is required to link such changes in membrane organization to improved contractility. The link between cellular and whole heart contractility is not direct because whole heart contraction is modified by a large number of factors not relevant to the single cell. Several studies show evidence that LVAD therapy enhances the ejection fraction,[5,8] suggesting improved whole heart function.

Cytoskeletal, Sarcomeric, and Membrane Proteins

LVAD therapy alters the expression of multiple sarcomeric, cytoskeletal, and linker proteins, suggesting an important role of these molecules in the process of reverse remodeling and possibly cardiac recovery (**Fig. 8**).[46–49] de Jonge and colleagues[50] demonstrated that the disrupted cellular cytoskeletal architecture observed in heart failure recovers to some extent after LVAD therapy (involving several proteins, including actin, tropomyosin, troponin T, and troponin C). A key molecular subset is the cell adhesion molecules,

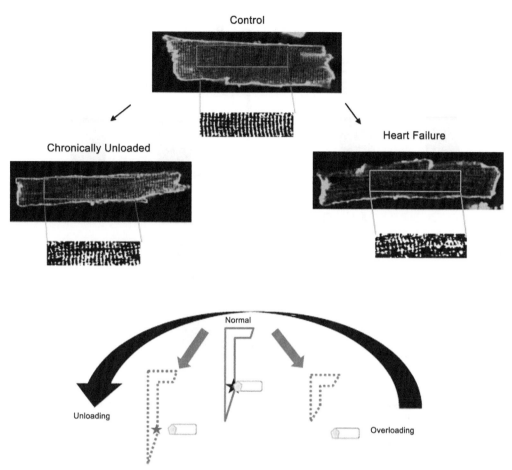

Fig. 6. The transverse tubules of failing rat hearts undergo reverse remodeling during mechanical unloading. The transverse tubules are essential for excitation-contraction coupling. They are lost in heart failure (preliminary work suggests they undergo reverse remodeling during mechanical unloading). (*From* Ibrahim M, Gorelik J, Yacoub M, et al. The structure and function of cardiac T-Tubules in health and disease. Proc Biol Sci 2011;278: 2714–23; with permission.)

the integrins.[51] These molecules span the membrane and link the ECM with the cytoskeleton. As such, they play an important role in mechanosensation and cell signaling. LVADs seem to induce recovery at multiple levels in the integrin pathway, which is disrupted in heart failure.[49] Whether this molecular recovery restores mechanosensation and the diverse actions of integrins is not yet known.

Myocardial and Subcellular Beta-Adrenergic System

One of the major regulators of cellular and myocardial contractility is the beta-adrenergic system, which is impaired in heart failure. The subcellular domains of different beta-adrenergic signaling pathways, which normally are spatially segregated, have recently been shown to be more globalized in failing cells compared with healthy cells in an animal model.[52] There is evidence that

mechanical unloading restores the membrane ultrastructure in animal models, which may result in relocalization of the cyclic adenosine monophosphate (cAMP) response to beta-adrenergic signaling, but this requires further experimental evidence.[39] At the whole-cell level, LVADs enhance the beta-adrenergic response of the myocardium, by increased receptor density[53] and by improved localization of beta receptors (**Fig. 9**).[54]

Metabolism

Mitochondrial and metabolic properties are major determinants of cardiac function, which is impaired in heart failure.[55] There is evidence that LVADs, apart from their dramatic effect in reducing cardiac workload, also induce reverse remodeling of metabolic and mitochondrial function in heart failure. This is mediated in part by restored respiratory capacity of mitochondria in heart failure and

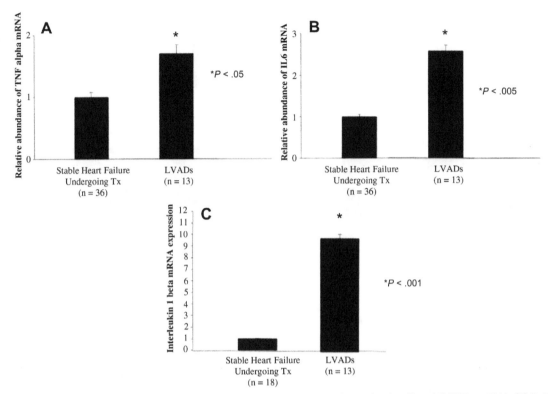

Fig. 7. Changes in elements of the innate immune system during mechanical unloading. (*A*) TNF-α mRNA, (*B*) IL-6 mRNA, and (*C*) IL-1β mRNA expression in LVAD candidates compared with stable patients with heart failure undergoing heart transplantation. (*From* Birks EJ, Felkin LE, Banner NR, et al. Increased toll-like receptor 4 in the myocardium of patients requiring left ventricular assist devices. J Heart Lung Transplant 2004;23:228–35; with permssion.)

by enhanced endogenous nitric oxide regulation of mitochondrial function.[56]

Apoptosis and Cell Regeneration

Heart failure is associated with increased apoptosis, which reduces cell numbers substantially. There is evidence that the enhanced cell death of heart failure is reversed by LVAD support, which increases the expression of the antiapoptotic proteins FasExo6Del,[57] BCL-XL levels,[58] and BCL-2[59]; and decreases markers of cellular apoptosis.[60]

Evidence showing that cardiomyocyte division occurs in response to cardiac injury[61,62] and the discovery of endogenous cardiac stem pools[63–65] may suggest that the myocardium is theoretically capable of regeneration under conditions of stress. The favorable environment during LVAD support, which improves the neurohormonal environment by reducing plasma adrenaline, noradrenaline, renin, aldosterone, and vasopressin[66]; as well as Atrial and B-type natriuretic peptide plasma levels,[67] could promote conditions for cardiac regeneration. Wohlschlaeger and colleagues[68] recently showed

a dramatic halving of mean cardiomyocyte DNA and a doubling of diploid cardiomyocytes, together with significant decrease in the number of polyploid cardiomyocytes (**Fig. 10**).[69,70] These results may imply that LVAD therapy promotes cardiomyocyte cell division.

IGF-1 mRNA levels are elevated at time of explantation of LVAD in patients treated with the Harefield protocol, suggesting elevated IGF-1 levels may be important in promoting recovery.[71] In experimental models of heart failure, IGF-1 administration improves function.[72,73] IGF-1 displays antiapoptotic properties[74] and promotes hypertrophy in skeletal[75,76] and cardiac muscle.[77,78]

The Architecture of Genetic and Protein Level Changes During LVAD Support

During LVAD support, there are changes at multiple genetic and protein levels, including changes to the expression of a large number of proteins and their posttranscriptional regulation.[79] MicroRNAs are small RNA sequences that do not code for protein directly, but can alter patterns of translation by binding with coding RNA sequences

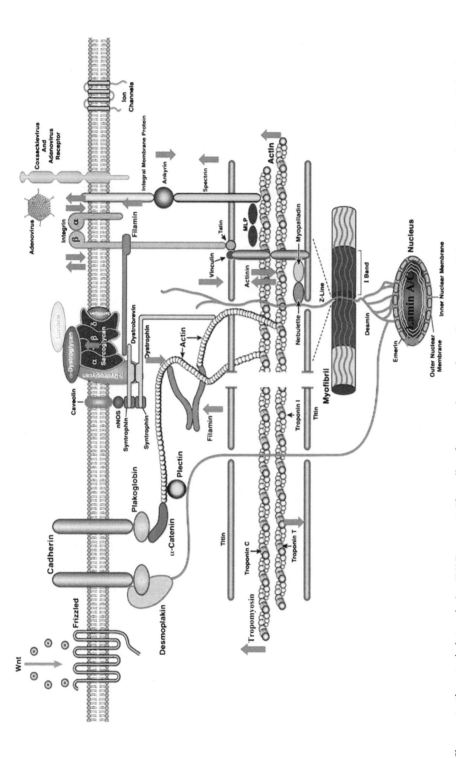

Fig. 8. Changes to the cytoskeleton during LVAD support. The cell surface membrane of a cardiomyocyte with its dense concentration of cytoskeletal proteins. The cytoskeleton provides mechanical support and is responsible for the transduction of several signals, including external mechanical load. The arrows depict the direction of changes in specific cytoskeletal proteins between the time of implantation and explantation. Changes occur in both sarcomeric and nonsarcomeric cytoskeletal components. MLP, muscle LIM protein. (*From* Birks EJ, Hall JL, Barton PJ et al. Gene profiling changes in cytoskeletal proteins during clinical recovery after left ventricular-assist device support. Circulation 2005;112:I57–64; with permission.)

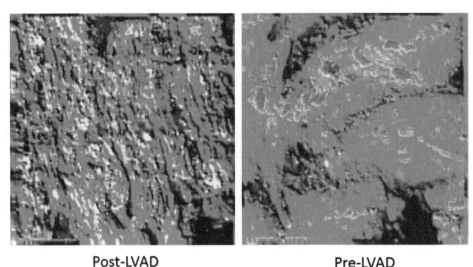

Post-LVAD   Pre-LVAD

Fig. 9. Changes to beta receptor localization in human myocardium before and after LVAD support. A pair of volume-rendered images in which beta-adrenergic receptors are visualized. The left panel is an explant sample (post-LVAD) and is compared with the right panel, a sample of panel of tissue at the time of LVAD implant (pre-LVAD) demonstrating the homogeneous versus clumped pattern of the receptors in the pre-LVAD tissue. This pattern is also seen with alpha receptors, as well as the receptors localized close to vascular elements and in extracellular spaces. Beta Adrenoceptor (βAR) numbers in this particular pair are 10,921 explant versus 3908 implant. (*From* Bick RJ, Grigore AM, Poindexter BJ, et al. Left ventricular unloading with an assist device results in receptor relocalization as well as increased beta-adrenergic receptor numbers: are these changes indications for outcome? J Card Surg 2005;20:332–6; with permission.)

and by influencing the pattern of protein expression. MicroRNA patterns appear to be normalized by LVAD therapy and could be a more sensitive marker for reverse remodeling than changes in gene expression.[80]

ECM

The ECM is a dynamic support architecture of multiple components influenced by both heart failure and LVAD therapy. Some studies show that LVAD therapy increases fibrosis,[81–85] and others show the opposite.[5,67,86–88] Apart from the content of collagen, the degree of collagen cross-linking is also important in determining the stiffness and, therefore, filling properties of the LV. Klotz and colleagues[81] showed that collagen cross-linking increased after LVAD therapy with consequent increase in myocardial stiffness. Bruggink and colleagues[89] demonstrated a biphasic response with initial increase in fibrosis followed by a subsequent regression with prolonged LVAD therapy. The molecular mechanisms governing the changes in collagen content and quality during heart failure and LVAD support include matrix metalloproteinases (MMPs), which degrade collagen, and their inhibitory regulators, the tissue inhibitors of metalloproteinases (TIMPs).

The fact that LVADs reduce the MMP1 to TIMP1 ratio has been reported with LVAD use in a DCM population. This results in enhanced LV collagen cross-linking and increased myocardial stiffness.[81] The degree of myocardial fibrosis[83,84] and profibrotic marker protein expression[90] at the point of LVAD implantation may predict the likelihood of cardiac recovery.

Pharmacologic blockade of the renin-angiotensin-aldosterone system in heart failure is known to decrease cardiac fibrosis, with associated improvements in mortality.[91] Klotz and colleagues[92] have shown that pharmacologic angiotensin-converting enzyme inhibition depresses the typical increase in total collagen levels and collagen cross-linking observed during LVAD therapy, which may enhance the rate of cardiac recovery. These changes are confined to the LV, indicating they arise due to mechanical unloading, not because of changes to the levels of circulating factors. Changes in other elements of the ECM including elastins, glycosaminoglycans, and their signaling molecules remain to be discovered.

Nonmyocyte Cells Populations

Multiple nonmyocyte populations have been under-investigated elements. They are activated in disease and during LVAD therapy and include the fibroblasts and endothelial cells. Importantly, the fibroblasts can influence cardiomyocyte structure and function and may be load-sensitive.[93] The

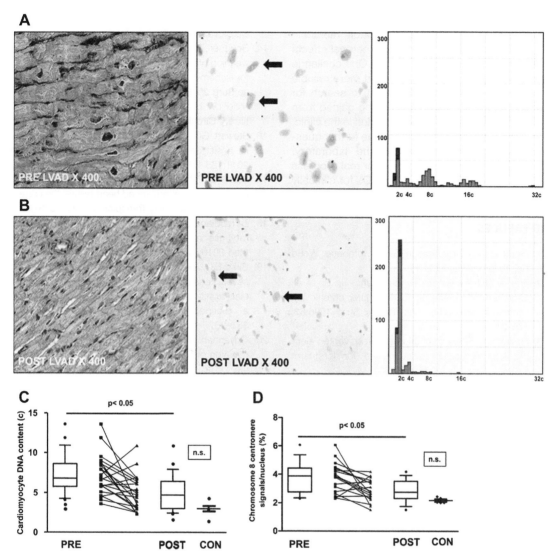

Fig. 10. Changes to cellular DNA content after LVAD support in humans. (*A, left*) Histologic specimen of the myocardium in heart failure. Note the enlarged cardiomyocytes with large hyperchromatic nuclei. (*A, middle*) Cell separation of myocardium in heart failure. Single hyperchromatic nuclei (Feulgen stain). (*A, right*) DNA image cytometry in heart failure showing increased numbers of cardiomyocytes with a genome greater than 2 c (*A*). (*B, left*) Histologic specimen of the same myocardium after mechanical support. Cardiomyocyte nuclei are smaller, and the nuclei are less hyperchromatic. (*B, middle*) Cell separation of myocardium after LVAD. Single smaller cardiomyocyte nuclei (Feulgen stain). (*B, right*) DNA cytometry showing decreased numbers of polyploid cardiomyocytes. (*C*) Significant decrease in the cardiomyocyte DNA content after unloading measured on isolated single cardiomyocyte nuclei by optical DNA cytometry. Unloaded and control hearts do not differ significantly in their DNA content, suggesting a decrease to physiologic DNA content. (*D*) To verify data obtained from optical DNA cytometry, the DNA content of paired myocardial samples was investigated by in situ hybridization with probes against the centromeres of chromosome 8. A significant decrease in centromeric signals after unloading was noted. (*From* Wohlschlaeger J, Levkau B, Brockhoff G et al. Hemodynamic support by left ventricular assist devices reduces cardiomyocyte DNA content in the failing human heart. Circulation 2010;121:989–96; with permission.)

fibroblasts are much more than mere collagen factories,[94] acting as sentinel cells regulating the immune system[95] and acting as regulators of the ECM in response to load.[93] Their role during LVAD support is a major topic for future studies.

SUMMARY AND FUTURE DIRECTIONS

The effort to understand the clinical pattern of BTR and its biologic mechanisms has substantially enhanced our knowledge of the mechanisms of heart failure and reverse remodeling, but there are many challenges remaining. Mechanistic changes at all the levels described probably interact in a complex network[96] where combinatorial effects determine the final clinical picture. One challenge is to develop cheaper, smaller, and more reliable devices and to enhance the effort to search for cardiac recovery. The understanding gained from laboratory studies needs to be applied in the clinic. The clinical experience will then raise further questions needing investigation in the laboratory. These efforts must be integrated for real progress in the long-term goal of using LVADs for clinically relevant BTR.

REFERENCES

1. World Health Organisation Global Infobase. World Health Organisation; 2011.
2. Frazier OH, Benedict CR, Radovancevic B, et al. Improved left ventricular function after chronic left ventricular unloading. Ann Thorac Surg 1996;62: 675–81.
3. Frazier OH. First use of an untethered, vented electric left ventricular assist device for long-term support. Circulation 1994;89:2908–14.
4. Mann DL, Willerson JT. Left ventricular assist devices and the failing heart: a bridge to recovery, a permanent assist device, or a bridge too far? Circulation 1998;98:2367–9.
5. Maybaum S, Mancini D, Xydas S, et al. Cardiac improvement during mechanical circulatory support: a prospective multicenter study of the LVAD Working Group. Circulation 2007;115:2497–505.
6. Mancini DM, Beniaminovitz A, Levin H, et al. Low incidence of myocardial recovery after left ventricular assist device implantation in patients with chronic heart failure. Circulation 1998;98:2383–9.
7. Yacoub MH. A novel strategy to maximize the efficacy of left ventricular assist devices as a bridge to recovery. Eur Heart J 2001;22:534–40.
8. Birks EJ, Tansley PD, Hardy J, et al. Left ventricular assist device and drug therapy for the reversal of heart failure. N Engl J Med 2006;355:1873–84.
9. Yacoub MH, Terracciano CM. The Holy Grail of LVAD-induced reversal of severe chronic heart failure: the need for integration. Eur Heart J 2011; 32:1052–4.
10. Fatkin D, Otway R, Richmond Z. Genetics of dilated cardiomyopathy. Heart Fail Clin 2010;6:129–40.
11. Yusuf SW, Ilias-Khan NA, Durand JB. Chemotherapy-induced cardiomyopathy. Expert Rev Cardiovasc Ther 2011;9:231–43.
12. Abboud J, Murad Y, Chen-Scarabelli C, et al. Peripartum cardiomyopathy: a comprehensive review. Int J Cardiol 2007;118:295–303.
13. Unosawa S, Hata M, Sezai A, et al. Successful recovery using surgical intervention to treat ischemic cardiomyopathy and cardiogenic shock. Ann Thorac Cardiovasc Surg 2010;16:52–4.
14. Beurtheret S, Mordant P, Pavie A, et al. Successful weaning of a left ventricular assist device implanted for ischemic heart failure. Interact Cardiovasc Thorac Surg 2010;11:507–9.
15. Miller LW. Left ventricular assist devices are underutilized. Circulation 2011;123:1552–8.
16. Stewart GC, Stevenson LW. Keeping left ventricular assist device acceleration on track. Circulation 2011;123:1559–68.
17. Stevenson LW, Pagani FD, Young JB, et al. INTERMACS profiles of advanced heart failure: the current picture. J Heart Lung Transplant 2009;28:535–41.
18. Terracciano CM, Miller LW, Yacoub MH. Contemporary use of ventricular assist devices. Annu Rev Med 2010;61:255–70.
19. Birks EJ, George RS, Hedger M, et al. Reversal of severe heart failure with a continuous-flow left ventricular assist device and pharmacological therapy: a prospective study. Circulation 2011;123(4): 381–90.
20. Oriyanhan W, Tsuneyoshi H, Nishina T, et al. Determination of optimal duration of mechanical unloading for failing hearts to achieve bridge to recovery in a rat heterotopic heart transplantation model. J Heart Lung Transplant 2007;26:16–23.
21. Dalby MC, Banner NR, Tansley P, et al. Left ventricular function during support with an asynchronous pulsatile left ventricular assist device. J Heart Lung Transplant 2003;22:292–300.
22. George RS, Yacoub MH, Tasca G, et al. Hemodynamic and echocardiographic responses to acute interruption of left ventricular assist device support: relevance to assessment of myocardial recovery. J Heart Lung Transplant 2007;26:967–73.
23. Kinoshita M, Takano H, Taenaka Y, et al. Cardiac disuse atrophy during LVAD pumping. ASAIO Trans 1988;34:208–12.
24. Soppa GK, Lee J, Stagg MA, et al. Prolonged mechanical unloading reduces myofilament sensitivity to calcium and sarcoplasmic reticulum calcium uptake leading to contractile dysfunction. J Heart Lung Transplant 2008;27:882–9.
25. Ibrahim M, Al Masri A, Navaratnarajah M, et al. Prolonged mechanical unloading affects cardiomyocyte excitation-contraction coupling, transverse-tubule structure, and the cell surface. FASEB J 2010;24: 3321–9.
26. Soppa GK, Smolenski RT, Latif N, et al. Effects of chronic administration of clenbuterol on function and metabolism of adult rat cardiac muscle. Am J Physiol Heart Circ Physiol 2005;288:H1468–76.
27. Siedlecka U, Arora M, Kolettis T, et al. Effects of clenbuterol on contractility and Ca2+ homeostasis of isolated rat ventricular myocytes. Am J Physiol Heart Circ Physiol 2008;295:H1917–26.

28. Barton PJ, Bhavsar PK, Felkin LE, et al. Morphological and molecular effects of clenbuterol on cardiac myocytes - role of IGF-1 [abstract]. J Heart Lung Transplant 2004;23:S53.

29. Frazier OH, Myers TJ. Left ventricular assist system as a bridge to myocardial recovery. Ann Thorac Surg 1999;68:734–41.

30. Dandel M, Weng Y, Siniawski H, et al. Prediction of cardiac stability after weaning from left ventricular assist devices in patients with idiopathic dilated cardiomyopathy. Circulation 2008;118:S94–105.

31. Hetzer R, Muller JH, Weng YG, et al. Midterm follow-up of patients who underwent removal of a left ventricular assist device after cardiac recovery from end-stage dilated cardiomyopathy. J Thorac Cardiovasc Surg 2000;120:843–53.

32. Rose EA, Gelijns AC, Moskowitz AJ, et al. Long-term mechanical left ventricular assistance for end-stage heart failure. N Engl J Med 2001;345:1435–43.

33. Dipla K, Mattiello JA, Jeevanandam V, et al. Myocyte recovery after mechanical circulatory support in humans with end-stage heart failure. Circulation 1998; 97:2316–22.

34. Terracciano CM, Hardy J, Birks EJ, et al. Clinical recovery from end-stage heart failure using left-ventricular assist device and pharmacological therapy correlates with increased sarcoplasmic reticulum calcium content but not with regression of cellular hypertrophy. Circulation 2004;109:2263–5.

35. Zafeiridis A, Jeevanandam V, Houser SR, et al. Regression of cellular hypertrophy after left ventricular assist device support. Circulation 1998;98:656–62.

36. Madigan JD, Barbone A, Choudhri AF, et al. Time course of reverse remodeling of the left ventricle during support with a left ventricular assist device. J Thorac Cardiovasc Surg 2001;121:902–8.

37. Bers DM. Altered cardiac myocyte Ca regulation in heart failure. Physiology (Bethesda) 2006;21:380–7.

38. Crossman DJ, Ruygrok PR, Soeller C, et al. Changes in the organization of excitation-contraction coupling structures in failing human heart. PLoS One 2011;6:e17901.

39. Ibrahim M, Navaratnarajah M, Siedlecka U, et al. Mechanical unloading of failing hearts normalises calcium-induced calcium release by reverse remodelling of the T-Tubule system [abstract]. Circulation 2010;122:A17308.

40. Birks EJ, Felkin LE, Banner NR, et al. Increased toll-like receptor 4 in the myocardium of patients requiring left ventricular assist devices. J Heart Lung Transplant 2004;23:228–35.

41. Birks EJ, Latif N, Owen V, et al. Quantitative myocardial cytokine expression and activation of the apoptotic pathway in patients who require left ventricular assist devices. Circulation 2001;104:I233–240.

42. Yamagishi T, Oshima K, Mohara J, et al. Cytokine induction owing to LVAD support in canine models. Transplant Proc 1999;31:1992–3.

43. Drakos SG, Terrovitis JV, Nanas JN, et al. Reverse electrophysiologic remodeling after cardiac mechanical unloading for end-stage nonischemic cardiomyopathy. Ann Thorac Surg 2011;91:764–9.

44. Harding JD, Piacentino V III, Gaughan JP, et al. Electrophysiological alterations after mechanical circulatory support in patients with advanced cardiac failure. Circulation 2001;104:1241–7.

45. Ibrahim M, Gorelik J, Yacoub M, et al. The structure and function of cardiac T-Tubules in health and disease. Proceedings of the Royal Society, Series B 2011. Proc Biol Sci 2011;278(1719):2714–23.

46. Margulies KB, Matiwala S, Cornejo C, et al. Mixed messages: transcription patterns in failing and recovering human myocardium. Circ Res 2005;96:592–9.

47. Vatta M, Stetson SJ, Perez-Verdia A, et al. Molecular remodelling of dystrophin in patients with end-stage cardiomyopathies and reversal in patients on assistance-device therapy. Lancet 2002;359:936–41.

48. Latif N, Yacoub MH, George R, et al. Changes in sarcomeric and non-sarcomeric cytoskeletal proteins and focal adhesion molecules during clinical myocardial recovery after left ventricular assist device support. J Heart Lung Transplant 2007;26:230–5.

49. Hall JL, Birks EJ, Grindle S, et al. Molecular signature of recovery following combination left ventricular assist device (LVAD) support and pharmacologic therapy. Eur Heart J 2007;28:613–27.

50. de Jonge N, van Wichen DF, Schipper ME, et al. Left ventricular assist device in end-stage heart failure: persistence of structural myocyte damage after unloading. An immunohistochemical analysis of the contractile myofilaments. J Am Coll Cardiol 2002; 39:963–9.

51. Kanchanawong P, Shtengel G, Pasapera AM, et al. Nanoscale architecture of integrin-based cell adhesions. Nature 2010;468:580–4.

52. Nikolaev VO, Moshkov A, Lyon AR, et al. Beta2-adrenergic receptor redistribution in heart failure changes cAMP compartmentation. Science 2010; 327:1653–7.

53. Ogletree-Hughes ML, Stull LB, Sweet WE, et al. Mechanical unloading restores beta-adrenergic responsiveness and reverses receptor downregulation in the failing human heart. Circulation 2001; 104:881–6.

54. Bick RJ, Grigore AM, Poindexter BJ, et al. Left ventricular unloading with an assist device results in receptor relocalization as well as increased beta-adrenergic receptor numbers: are these changes indications for outcome? J Card Surg 2005;20:332–6.

55. Neubauer S. The failing heart–an engine out of fuel. N Engl J Med 2007;356:1140–51.

56. Mital S, Loke KE, Addonizio LJ, et al. Left ventricular assist device implantation augments nitric oxide dependent control of mitochondrial respiration in failing human hearts. J Am Coll Cardiol 2000;36:1897–902.

57. Bartling B, Milting H, Schumann H, et al. Myocardial gene expression of regulators of myocyte apoptosis and myocyte calcium homeostasis during hemodynamic unloading by ventricular assist devices in patients with end-stage heart failure. Circulation 1999;100:II216–23.

58. Milting H, Bartling B, Schumann H, et al. Altered levels of mRNA of apoptosis-mediating genes after mid-term mechanical ventricular support in dilative cardiomyopathy–first results of the Halle Assist Induced Recovery Study (HAIR). Thorac Cardiovasc Surg 1999;47:48–50.

59. Francis GS, Anwar F, Bank AJ, et al. Apoptosis, Bcl-2, and proliferating cell nuclear antigen in the failing human heart: observations made after implantation of left ventricular assist device. J Card Fail 1999;5:308–15.

60. Baba HA, Grabellus F, August C, et al. Reversal of metallothionein expression is different throughout the human myocardium after prolonged left-ventricular mechanical support. J Heart Lung Transplant 2000;19:668–74.

61. Beltrami AP, Urbanek K, Kajstura J, et al. Evidence that human cardiac myocytes divide after myocardial infarction. N Engl J Med 2001;344:1750–7.

62. Engel FB, Hsieh PC, Lee RT, et al. FGF1/p38 MAP kinase inhibitor therapy induces cardiomyocyte mitosis, reduces scarring, and rescues function after myocardial infarction. Proc Natl Acad Sci U S A 2006;103:15546–51.

63. Hosoda T, Kajstura J, Leri A, et al. Mechanisms of myocardial regeneration. Circ J 2010;74:13–7.

64. Leri A, Kajstura J, Anversa P. Cardiac stem cells and mechanisms of myocardial regeneration. Physiol Rev 2005;85:1373–416.

65. Urbanek K, Torella D, Sheikh F, et al. Myocardial regeneration by activation of multipotent cardiac stem cells in ischemic heart failure. Proc Natl Acad Sci U S A 2005;102:8692–7.

66. Klotz S, Burkhoff D, Garrelds IM, et al. The impact of left ventricular assist device-induced left ventricular unloading on the myocardial renin-angiotensin-aldosterone system: therapeutic consequences? Eur Heart J 2009;30:805–12.

67. Thompson LO, Skrabal CA, Loebe M, et al. Plasma neurohormone levels correlate with left ventricular functional and morphological improvement in LVAD patients. J Surg Res 2005;123:25–32.

68. Adler CP, Sandritter W. Alterations of substances (DNA, myoglobin, myosin, protein) in experimentally induced cardiac hypertrophy and under the influence of drugs (isoproterenol, cytostatics, strophanthin). Basic Res Cardiol 1980;75:126–38.

69. Sandritter W, Adler CP. Polyploidization of heart muscle nuclei as a prerequisite for heart growth and numerical hyperplasia in heart hypertrophy. Recent Adv Stud Cardiac Struct Metab 1976;12:115–27.

70. Wohlschlaeger J, Levkau B, Brockhoff G, et al. Hemodynamic support by left ventricular assist devices reduces cardiomyocyte DNA content in the failing human heart. Circulation 2010;121:989–96.

71. Barton PJ, Felkin LE, Birks EJ, et al. Myocardial insulin-like growth factor-I gene expression during recovery from heart failure after combined left ventricular assist device and clenbuterol therapy. Circulation 2005;112:I46–50.

72. Duerr RL, Huang S, Miraliakbar HR, et al. Insulin-like growth factor-1 enhances ventricular hypertrophy and function during the onset of experimental cardiac failure. J Clin Invest 1995;95:619–27.

73. Duerr RL, McKirnan MD, Gim RD, et al. Cardiovascular effects of insulin-like growth factor-1 and growth hormone in chronic left ventricular failure in the rat. Circulation 1996;93:2188–96.

74. Li Q, Li B, Wang X, et al. Overexpression of insulin-like growth factor-1 in mice protects from myocyte death after infarction, attenuating ventricular dilation, wall stress, and cardiac hypertrophy. J Clin Invest 1997;100:1991–9.

75. Musaro A. Growth factor enhancement of muscle regeneration: a central role of IGF-1. Arch Ital Biol 2005;143:243–8.

76. Pelosi L, Giacinti C, Nardis C, et al. Local expression of IGF-1 accelerates muscle regeneration by rapidly modulating inflammatory cytokines and chemokines. FASEB J 2007;21:1393–402.

77. Santini MP, Tsao L, Monassier L, et al. Enhancing repair of the mammalian heart. Circ Res 2007;100:1732–40.

78. Welch S, Plank D, Witt S, et al. Cardiac-specific IGF-1 expression attenuates dilated cardiomyopathy in tropomodulin-overexpressing transgenic mice. Circ Res 2002;90:641–8.

79. Milting H, Scholz C, Arusoglu L, et al. Selective upregulation of beta1-adrenergic receptors and dephosphorylation of troponin I in end-stage heart failure patients supported by ventricular assist devices. J Mol Cell Cardiol 2006;41:441–50.

80. Matkovich SJ, Van Booven DJ, Youker KA, et al. Reciprocal regulation of myocardial microRNAs and messenger RNA in human cardiomyopathy and reversal of the microRNA signature by biomechanical support. Circulation 2009;119:1263–71.

81. Klotz S, Foronjy RF, Dickstein ML, et al. Mechanical unloading during left ventricular assist device support increases left ventricular collagen cross-linking and myocardial stiffness. Circulation 2005;112:364–74.

82. Li YY, Feng Y, McTiernan CF, et al. Downregulation of matrix metalloproteinases and reduction in collagen damage in the failing human heart after support with left ventricular assist devices. Circulation 2001;104:1147–52.

83. Matsumiya G, Monta O, Fukushima N, et al. Who would be a candidate for bridge to recovery during prolonged mechanical left ventricular support in idiopathic dilated cardiomyopathy? J Thorac Cardiovasc Surg 2005;130:699–704.

84. Saito S, Matsumiya G, Sakaguchi T, et al. Cardiac fibrosis and cellular hypertrophy decrease the degree of reverse remodeling and improvement in cardiac function during left ventricular assist. J Heart Lung Transplant 2010;29:672–9.

85. Drakos SG, Kfoury AG, Hammond EH, et al. Impact of mechanical unloading on microvasculature and associated central remodeling features of the failing human heart. J Am Coll Cardiol 2010;56:382–91.

86. Akgul A, Skrabal CA, Thompson LO, et al. Role of mast cells and their mediators in failing myocardium under mechanical ventricular support. J Heart Lung Transplant 2004;23:709–15.

87. Bruckner BA, Stetson SJ, Perez-Verdia A, et al. Regression of fibrosis and hypertrophy in failing myocardium following mechanical circulatory support. J Heart Lung Transplant 2001;20:457–64.

88. Thohan V, Stetson SJ, Nagueh SF, et al. Cellular and hemodynamics responses of failing myocardium to continuous flow mechanical circulatory support using the DeBakey-Noon left ventricular assist device: a comparative analysis with pulsatile-type devices. J Heart Lung Transplant 2005;24:566–75.

89. Bruggink AH, van Oosterhout MF, De JN, et al. Reverse remodeling of the myocardial extracellular matrix after prolonged left ventricular assist device support follows a biphasic pattern. J Heart Lung Transplant 2006;25:1091–8.

90. Felkin LE, Lara-Pezzi E, George R, et al. Expression of extracellular matrix genes during myocardial recovery from heart failure after left ventricular assist device support. J Heart Lung Transplant 2009;28:117–22.

91. Arnold JM, Yusuf S, Young J, et al. Prevention of Heart Failure in Patients in the Heart Outcomes Prevention Evaluation (HOPE) Study. Circulation 2003;107:1284–90.

92. Klotz S, Danser AH, Foronjy RF, et al. The impact of angiotensin-converting enzyme inhibitor therapy on the extracellular collagen matrix during left ventricular assist device support in patients with end-stage heart failure. J Am Coll Cardiol 2007;49:1166–74.

93. MacKenna D, Summerour SR, Villarreal FJ. Role of mechanical factors in modulating cardiac fibroblast function and extracellular matrix synthesis. Cardiovasc Res 2000;46:257–63.

94. Camelliti P, Borg TK, Kohl P. Structural and functional characterisation of cardiac fibroblasts. Cardiovasc Res 2005;65:40–51.

95. Smith RS, Smith TJ, Blieden TM, et al. Fibroblasts as sentinel cells. Synthesis of chemokines and regulation of inflammation. Am J Pathol 1997;151:317–22.

96. Egerstedt M. Complex networks: degrees of control. Nature 2011;473:158–9.

Editorial Comment on "Bridge to Recovery: What Remains to be Discovered?"

John A. Elefteriades, MD

KEY CONCEPTS

That myocardial recovery can occur in some patients after LVAD support has been abundantly demonstrated by Professor Magdi Yacoub and his group (the authors of "Bridge to Recovery: What Remains to be Discovered?") and documented in an extraordinary panel of publications, which describe not only the clinical phenomena but also their fundamental molecular and structural underpinnings.

STRENGTHS

There is no doubt that recovery can and does occur. Guidelines are given for selection of patients, weaning patterns, and monitoring during and after weaning. Insights are provided on how (beneficial) reverse remodelling occurs pathophysiologically.

WEAKNESSES

Despite the remarkable efforts to characterize and understand bridge to recovery, it remains to be determined with complete clarity which patients should have an LVAD, what type should be used, how the device should be programmed to promote recovery, how to augment recovery pharmacologically, how to monitor recovery, what criteria to satisfy before recovery, and how to ensure a relapse-free recovery.

Section of Cardiac Surgery, Yale University School of Medicine, Boardman 2, 333 Cedar Street, New Haven, CT 06510, USA

E-mail address: john.elefteriades@yale.edu

Cardiol Clin 29 (2011) 549
doi:10.1016/j.ccl.2011.07.006
0733-8651/11/$ – see front matter

cardiology.theclinics.com

Tips on Tuning Each Device: Technical Pearls

Hiroo Takayama, MD, Jonathan A. Yang, MD,
Yoshifumi Naka, MD, PhD*

KEYWORDS

- Implantation technique • HeartMate XVE • HeartMate II
- HeartWare • DuraHeart

Significant improvement has been made in ventricular assist device (VAD) technology, and this has led to an expanding use of this technology in various scenarios in which a patient suffers from end-stage heart failure (HF). VADs work as an extra pump to support circulation. These devices consist of an inflow, through which the blood is drained from the native circulation; a pump; and an outflow, through which the blood is returned back to the patient. Although simple in concept, successful implementation of this technology requires appropriate experience and substantial up-to-date knowledge regarding best practices for surgical technique and management, which go far beyond just understanding the basic mechanics. One of the most important aspects of patient care associated with VADs is the surgical technique at implantation. Technical pitfalls that have been identified over the years are described for each device with a focus on implantable long-term left VADs (LVADs). In addition to the devices discussed in this review, there are other devices that are or will soon be undergoing clinical trial but are beyond the scope of this review.

GENERAL SURGICAL TECHNIQUE OF LONG-TERM LVAD IMPLANTATION

It will be useful to describe the general technique of LVAD implantation because most of the steps are shared for many implantable LVADs.

A vertical midline incision is made with extension onto the abdominal wall. After standard median sternotomy, a pocket of an appropriate size is created in the preperitoneal space in the upper abdomen.[1] If the preperitoneal plane is very thin and attenuated, the posterior rectus sheath is entered and a plane superficial to this is developed. The device is positioned in the preperitoneal pocket, and the driveline is tunneled. After systemic heparinization, the patient is cannulated for cardiopulmonary bypass. If the hemodynamic status permits, the outflow graft anastomosis is performed off-pump using a partial occluding clamp placed on the ascending aorta. Cardiopulmonary bypass is initiated, and the left ventricle (LV) is decompressed by placing a vent through a stab wound at the LV apex. For reoperative LVAD implantation, the posterior pericardial space is dissected out just enough to elevate the apex to sew the inflow cuff (**Fig. 1**). As bleeding from this area can be significant after reoperative LVAD implantation, careful hemostasis is crucial. The LV apical core is excised with a specialized coring knife. Care must be taken when coring to avoid deviation into the septum or the lateral wall. Any excess trabeculations or myocardium that may obstruct the inflow cannula is excised, as well as ventricular intramural thrombus. The inflow cuff is secured to the edges of the core with 2-0 braided polyester sutures reinforced with felt pledgets and then attached to the inflow

Yoshifumi Naka receives consultant fee from Thoratec and DuraHeart. The other authors have nothing to disclose.
Department of Surgery, Columbia University Medical Center, Milstein Hospital Building, 7-435, 177 Fort Washington Avenue, New York, NY 10032, USA
* Corresponding author.
E-mail address: yn33@columbia.edu

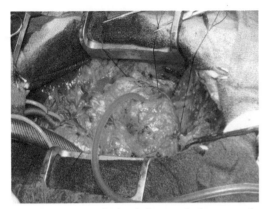

Fig. 1. Exposure of the left ventricular apex for reoperative LVAD implantation. The apex is elevated with several deep pericardial stitches. A vent is inserted through a stab wound at the apex for decompression.

cannula of the device. For fragile myocardium, this suture line is reinforced with a strip of Teflon felt (**Fig. 2**). The heart is allowed to fill with blood, and the device is deaired through a venting hole placed in the outflow graft. Evacuation of air is confirmed with transesophageal echocardiogram (TEE). The patient is then weaned from cardiopulmonary bypass, and the device is initiated.

PREPARATION FOR RESTERNOTOMY

Not just a small subset of patients with an LVAD requires another sternotomy for reasons such as heart transplantation or device exchange. Sternal reentry after a VAD implantation is challenging because development of dense adhesions around the heart and the device is usually the case. At the time of LVAD implantation, the surgeon is responsible for anticipating the possibility of a future cardiac operation. The same principles used

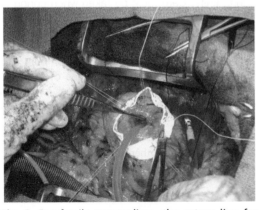

Fig. 2. For fragile myocardium, the suture line for inflow cuff placement is reinforced with a strip of Teflon felt.

during other cardiac surgery are followed for the prevention of postoperative bleeding and infectious complications, thus reducing the formation of adhesions.

In addition, to reduce the difficulty in performing repeat sternotomy, several measures are implemented in our program. Various membranes have been tried to protect the underlying cardiovascular structures on sternal reentry. We used to place a piece of thick polytetrafluoroethylene patch between the anterior surface of the heart and the sternum. However, this technique resulted in adhesions between the patch and the sternum, which can deceive surgeons at sternal reentry who perceive it to be the posterior plate of the sternum. In addition, the technique also creates tight adhesions with the heart. Thus, we abandoned this material as "a recipe for disasters." Until recently, the most commonly used material at our institution was a thin expanded polytetrafluoroethylene membrane. This pericardial substitute has been reported to be safe and effective in reducing the risk of sternal reentry for various types of cardiac reoperations, including those after VAD implantation, although in patients who underwent reoperation, the underlying epicardium and coronary vessels were sometimes obscured by a film of fine adhesions.[2,3] Another option is to use an extracellular matrix (ECM) membrane. Recently, with advancements in tissue engineering, elements of the ECM have gained increasing attention as crucial elements in maintaining the characteristics of 3-dimensional cardiac cell aggregates.[4] ECM, once regarded as merely a scaffold for developing tissue, plays an important role in providing essential signals that influence major intracellular pathways such as proliferation, differentiation, and cell metabolism. One of the synthetic ECM products, CorMatrix (CorMatrix Cardiovascular, Inc, Alpharetta, GA, USA), is made from sterilized and decellularized porcine small intestinal submucosa. When used to reconstruct pericardium, this product allows cells to infiltrate the ECM to remodel and form a new pericardial layer. The CorMatrix has gained attention and is increasingly used in clinical practice. We have used this product for pericardial reconstruction after a VAD implantation and have experienced its satisfactory antifibrotic property at subsequent VAD-explant heart transplantation (based on authors anecdotal clinical experience). The edge of the CorMatrix is secured to the edge of the opened pericardium with a 4-0 polypropylene running suture to cover the entire heart and inflow and outflow conduits. At reoperation, it is common to find some adhesions between this tissue and the underlying heart, but it is usually very easy to define the edge of the pericardium, and intrapericardial adhesions appear to be reduced compared with those with other materials such as an expanded polytetrafluoroethylene membrane.

In addition to placing a protective membrane, using a sealant material might reduce the formation of adhesions. Cannata and colleagues[5] reported a case in which a surgical sealant, CoSeal (Baxter Health care Corp, Fremont, CA, USA), was applied on the cardiac surface at LVAD implantation. At resternotomy for heart transplantation, surgical dissection of the LVAD was greatly facilitated by the presence of avascular loose adhesions. CoSeal is a sprayable polymeric matrix composed of 2 synthetic polyethylene glycols, originally developed and adopted as a surgical sealant for the control of bleeding from cardiovascular anastomoses.[6] An experimental model showed a significant reduction of adhesions after sternotomy and pericardiotomy in CoSeal-treated rabbits compared with controls.[7] Initial experience with CoSeal to prevent adhesions in pediatric cardiac surgery has also been promising.[8]

Injury of the outflow graft during sternal reentry creates a devastating situation. To avoid this situation on resternotomy, care should be taken during implantation to place the graft off midline, to the right side of the anterior mediastinum. This placement requires an outflow graft cut to the appropriate length; too short a graft results in midline positioning and too long a graft results in intrathoracic positioning or kinking. Expansion of the Dacron graft with pressurization needs to be taken into consideration in determining its length. The graft can also be covered with the graft remnant as another layer of protection.

CARDIAC STRUCTURAL PATHOLOGIES THAT REQUIRE SURGICAL CORRECTION

There are several anatomic pathologies that require special attention.

Significant semilunar valve regurgitation needs to be repaired during any type of mechanical circulatory support device insertion because it creates a recirculation circuit with the device. Perhaps more importantly, recent studies, including our own investigations, have shown a correlation between the development of aortic insufficiency (AI) and continuous flow (CF) LVAD support.[9,10] Implantable CF LVADs are currently the mainstay of LVAD therapy because of their reliability and superior performance compared with other technologies.[11,12] Long-term use, however, may lead to greater issues with AI. Thus, we currently do not tolerate any AI at the time of long-term CF LVAD implantation. The aortic valve is assessed with intraoperative TEE, and, if even trace AI is

found, the valve is repaired, whenever feasible, by suturing together the center of each leaflet (the node of Arantius) with a 4-0 polypropylene suture buttressed with small tissue pledgets (**Fig. 3**). The procedure requires aortic cross-clamp and cardioplegic arrest. The long-term outcomes of this strategy remain to be seen. This strategy is not applicable to other VADs, such as any short-term VADs or pulsatile flow (PF) LVADs, because of differences in duration of support or expected flow across the aortic valve. In these cases, AI is addressed only when it is moderate or more. When replacement is needed, a bioprosthesis is used.

Mechanical aortic valve prostheses can thrombose or become thrombogenic in the setting of LVAD support because of significantly decreased flow across the valve. Replacement with a bioprosthesis or closure with a patch needs to be performed.[13]

Other important anatomic abnormalities that require surgical correction at LVAD implantation include patent foramen ovale (PFO), tricuspid regurgitation (TR), and LV apical thrombus.

After LVAD implantation, the left atrial pressure could become lower than the right atrial pressure, especially in the setting of borderline right ventricle (RV) function. This pressure difference exacerbates right to left shunting through a PFO and can cause profound hypoxia.[14] Whenever intraoperative TEE with bubble study identifies a PFO, it is closed with bicaval cannulation. No cardiac arrest is required for this procedure. The LV is decompressed by placing a vent through the apex with the heart beating before the right atrium is opened. We also routinely ask the anesthesiologist to perform a TEE bubble study after LVAD placement to rule out a small PFO that might have been left undetected.

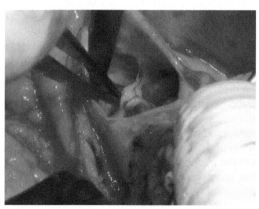

Fig. 3. Aortic valve repair is performed by suturing together the center of each leaflet (the node of Arantius) with a 4-0 polypropylene suture buttressed with small tissue pledgets.

Patients with HF have a high incidence of TR due to dilatation of the tricuspid annulus, RV dysfunction, and the presence of pacing leads. No consensus exists as to the appropriate indications of repair for TR.[13,15] However, we routinely repair significant TR at the time of LVAD implantation to maximize forward flow from the RV. The repair is usually readily accomplished by placing a ring, but additional repair techniques may be necessary for leaflet pathology created by pacing leads. No cardiac arrest is needed.

LV mural thrombi occur in one-third of Q wave acute myocardial infarction cases, 50% of LV aneurysms, and up to 18% of hearts with dilated cardiomyopathy.[16] Cardioplegic arrest might be required for removal of the LV thrombus to prevent systemic embolization.

TECHNICAL PERILS SPECIFIC TO DEVICES
HeartMate XVE

The HeartMate (HM) XVE (Thoratec Corp, Pleasanton, CA, USA) was the first LVAD that received Food and Drug Administration (FDA) approval for both bridge to transplant (BTT) and destination therapy (DT). This device generates PF through a pusher plate situated in a relatively large housing, which is placed in the anterior abdomen. Two 25-mm porcine valves are seated in the inflow and outflow arms. Because of the device's size and perhaps its pulsatility (generating higher systolic pressure compared with a CF pump), there may be more blood loss with its implantation compared with a CF LVAD implantation. A large pocket, necessary to accommodate the large pump, requires meticulous hemostasis of the soft tissue. We have also encountered unexpected postoperative bleeding from the distal portion of the left internal mammary artery because of erosion from the pulsatile motion of the inflow arm. Preemptive ligation of the artery might be considered if it is close to the inflow arm. The outflow graft of the HM XVE is larger than that of the HM II (Thoratec Corp, Pleasanton, CA, USA) (20 mm vs 14 mm). Oozing from the anastomosis between the graft and the ascending aorta creates a cumbersome situation. Our anastomotic technique is as follows: 4 mattress sutures of 4-0 polypropylene buttressed with small pledgets are placed and tied down at 4 corners, at the top and bottom apices and the midportion of each side of the aortotomy. The anastomosis is completed by running these sutures.

HM II

The CF of the HM II is driven by a small axial pump, which generates up to 10 L/min of blood flow.

There are only 2 bearings in the device, which makes this device more durable. The percutaneous driveline of this device is also significantly smaller than that of the HM XVE. This device has received FDA approval both for BTT and DT. A much smaller pocket is created. However, too small a pocket may distort the alignment at the LV apex between the long axis of the LV and the inflow cannula, which can promote occlusion or thrombus formation at the inflow site. The positioning of the driveline also needs attention. Any acute angulation should be avoided to prevent lead fracture. To decrease the risk of a driveline infection extending to the LVAD pocket, the driveline is tunneled through a long subcutaneous tract. The driveline is brought out of the skin through the first counterincision in the right upper quadrant and then through the second punched-out incision placed in the left upper quadrant (**Fig. 4**).

HeartWare LVAD

The HeartWare LVAD (HeartWare International, Inc, Framingham, MA, USA) is a centrifugal pump whose impeller is suspended within the housing without any mechanical contact by magnets and a hydrodynamic thrust bearing. This device can generate up to 10 L/min of flow. The result of a pivotal trial testing its feasibility for BTT use was reported at the American Heart Association 2010, demonstrating promising results. The device is currently undergoing a trial for DT use.

The distinct feature of the device is its small pump, which is directly incorporated into the inflow cuff, allowing intrapericardial placement. No creation of a pocket is needed. Several locations are proposed as a proper location for the inflow cannula. The recommendation from the

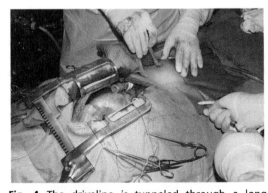

Fig. 4. The driveline is tunneled through a long subcutaneous tract. The driveline is brought out of the skin through the first counterincision in the right upper quadrant and then through the second punched-out incision placed in the left upper quadrant.

manufacture is slightly anterior to the LV apex, although the inflow cannula is commonly placed at the usual LV apex similar to other LVADs. The inflow cannula was originally designed to be inserted into the diaphragmatic surface of the heart. Gregoric and colleagues[17] reported that this original technique resulted in the optimal left ventricular position, with orientation of the inlet cannula parallel to the short axis of the LV and anterior to the papillary muscle insertion. A site for the sewing ring and core is selected at approximately one-third of the distance from the apex to the base of the heart and slightly lateral to the posterior descending artery. Another point, although not as important, is that it is recommended to create a core after the attachment of the sewing cuff to the LV. Because the rigid coring device requires certain experience for proper use, some investigators prefer to create the tract manually without the device. Too large a core must be avoided because it causes bleeding. The core tract must be slightly smaller than the inflow cannula for tight and hemostatic fit. Care should be taken in measuring the length of the outflow graft, which is significantly longer than other LVADs.

DuraHeart

The DuraHeart (Terumo Heart Inc, Ann Arbor, MI, USA) uses a centrifugal pump in which the impeller is magnetically levitated in the pump chamber, thereby generating blood flow without mechanical friction in the blood chamber. The pump is housed in a titanium enclosure that hermetically seals the electrical components against any blood or tissue contact. A surface treatment containing a heparin derivative is applied to the surfaces in contact with blood to reduce the risk of thrombus formation. Clinical experience has been accumulated mainly in Europe.[18] In 2007, the DuraHeart received CE mark approval in Europe for patients with end-stage HF and is currently undergoing clinical trial for BTT in the United States. The essences of the implantation technique are the same as those of other LVADs. The pitfalls of DuraHeart's implantation technique are focused on its small but relatively high-profile pump as well as the fixed angle of the inflow arm in relation to the pump. A generous preperitoneal pocket must be created to accommodate the pump. The preperitoneal pocket needs special attention to avoid inflow occlusion. A proper angulation of the inflow arm and its depth into the LV should be set before final fixation to the LV, and positioning of the tip of the inflow cannula in the LV is to be carefully assessed with TEE so that it does not point toward the septum or the lateral wall.

SUMMARY

Although the basic technique is relatively similar among the currently available devices, there are many subtle potential technical pitfalls for each device that could result in grave adverse events. It is not enough for implanting surgeons to be familiar with the recommended technique for each device, but experience with technical details and pitfalls should be shared among surgeons to improve outcomes.

REFERENCES

1. McCarthy PM, Wang N, Vargo R. Preperitoneal insertion of the HeartMate 1000 IP implantable left ventricular assist device. Ann Thorac Surg 1994; 57(3):634–7 [discussion: 637–8].
2. Leprince P, Rahmati M, Bonnet N, et al. Expanded polytetrafluoroethylene membranes to wrap surfaces of circulatory support devices in patients undergoing bridge to heart transplantation. Eur J Cardiothorac Surg 2001;19(3):302–6.
3. Jacobs JP, Iyer RS, Weston JS, et al. Expanded PTFE membrane to prevent cardiac injury during resternotomy for congenital heart disease. Ann Thorac Surg 1996;62(6):1778–82.
4. Akhyari P, Kamiya H, Haverich A, et al. Myocardial tissue engineering: the extracellular matrix. Eur J Cardiothorac Surg 2008;34(2):229–41.
5. Cannata A, Taglieri C, Russo CF, et al. Use of CoSeal in a patient with a left ventricular assist device. Ann Thorac Surg 2009;87(6):1956–8.
6. Glickman M, Gheissari A, Money S, et al. A polymeric sealant inhibits anastomotic suture hole bleeding more rapidly than gelfoam/thrombin: results of a randomized controlled trial. Arch Surg 2002;137(3): 326–31 [discussion: 332].
7. Marc Hendrikx M, Mees U, Hill AC, et al. Evaluation of a novel synthetic sealant for inhibition of cardiac adhesions and clinical experience in cardiac surgery procedures. Heart Surg Forum 2001;4(3):204–9 [discussion: 210].
8. Pace Napoleone C, Oppido G, Angeli E, et al. Resternotomy in pediatric cardiac surgery: CoSeal initial experience. Interact Cardiovasc Thorac Surg 2007; 6(1):21–3.
9. Pak SW, Uriel N, Takayama H, et al. Prevalence of de novo aortic insufficiency during long-term support with left ventricular assist devices. J Heart Lung Transplant 2010;29(10):1172–6.
10. Cowger J, Pagani FD, Haft JW, et al. The development of aortic insufficiency in left ventricular assist device-supported patients. Circ Heart Fail 2010; 3(6):668–74.
11. Slaughter MS, Rogers JG, Milano CA, et al. Advanced heart failure treated with continuous-flow

left ventricular assist device. N Engl J Med 2009; 361(23):2241–51.

12. Kirklin JK, Naftel DC, Kormos RL, et al. Third INTERMACS Annual Report: the evolution of destination therapy in the United States. J Heart Lung Transplant 2011;30(2):115–23.

13. Rao V, Slater JP, Edwards NM, et al. Surgical management of valvular disease in patients requiring left ventricular assist device support. Ann Thorac Surg 2001;71(5):1448–53.

14. Kapur NK, Conte JV, Resar JR. Percutaneous closure of patent foramen ovale for refractory hypoxemia after HeartMate II left ventricular assist device placement. J Invasive Cardiol 2007;19(9): E268–70.

15. Saeed D, Kidambi T, Shalli S, et al. Tricuspid valve repair with left ventricular assist device implantation: is it warranted? J Heart Lung Transplant 2011;30(5): 530–5.

16. Cregler LL. Antithrombotic therapy in left ventricular thrombosis and systemic embolism. Am Heart J 1992;123(4 Pt 2):1110–4.

17. Gregoric ID, Cohn WE, Frazier OH. Diaphragmatic implantation of the HeartWare ventricular assist device. J Heart Lung Transplant 2011;30(4):467–70.

18. Morshuis M, El-Banayosy A, Arusoglu L, et al. European experience of DuraHeart magnetically levitated centrifugal left ventricular assist system. Eur J Cardiothorac Surg 2009;35(6):1020–7 [discussion: 1027–28].

Editorial Comments on "Tips on 'Tuning' Each Device— Technical Pearls"

John A. Elefteriades, MD

KEY CONCEPTS

In "Tips on 'Tuning' Each Device—Technical Pearls," Dr Yoshifumi Naka and colleagues systematically review general principles and tips specific to each of several popular devices. This surgical guidance is immensely valuable, reflecting Dr Naka's extensive clinical experience.

STRENGTHS

As above.

WEAKNESSES

None.

Section of Cardiac Surgery, Yale University School of Medicine, Boardman 2, 333 Cedar Street, New Haven, CT 06510, USA
E-mail address: john.elefteriades@yale.edu

Cardiol Clin 29 (2011) 557
doi:10.1016/j.ccl.2011.07.010

The Future of Adult Cardiac Assist Devices: Novel Systems and Mechanical Circulatory Support Strategies

Carlo R. Bartoli, PhD[a], Robert D. Dowling, MD[b],*

KEYWORDS

- Heart failure • Left ventricular assist device (LVAD)
- Right ventricular assist device (RVAD)
- Total artificial heart (TAH) • Pulsatile flow
- Continuous flow • Full support • Partial support
- Mechanical circulatory support

Adult patients with advanced heart failure that is refractory to pharmacologic and electrical resynchronization therapies have a limited prognosis. For select patients, heart transplantation offers the best opportunity for long-term survival. However, the number of available donor hearts (~3500 annually worldwide) is inadequate to meet the needs of more than 30,000 patients listed for heart transplantation worldwide each year.[1] As a result, cardiac transplant waiting lists have the highest mortality (30%) of any of the solid organ waiting lists.[2] If a patient does receive a donor heart, chronic rejection and sequelae of long-term immunosuppression limit posttransplant survival to 55% at 10 years.[3] Furthermore, many patients are not considered for transplantation because of age, comorbidities, or even inadequate insurance coverage. As a result, more patients are being considered for destination therapy with a permanent, implantable cardiac assist device. In the past decade mechanical circulatory support therapies have emerged as a standard, long-term therapy for adult patients with advanced, intractable heart failure.

Currently, more than 20 novel cardiac assist devices are being developed or are in clinical trials, with nearly a dozen new systems ready to begin clinical trials before 2015.[4–18] Each device entails unique surgical and physiologic considerations and offers benefits and drawbacks for the patient and the physician. For example, currently available left ventricular assist devices (LVADs) require extensive surgery but can replace cardiac function. These "full-support" devices are reserved as a final treatment option only for patients with life-threatening heart failure. Consequently, physicians may be reluctant to refer less-sick patients for invasive, full-support LVAD therapy.

To expand the role of mechanical circulatory support for the treatment of heart failure, investigators and industry partners are miniaturizing LVADs for less-invasive and earlier therapy. Small devices that are designed to provide moderate or "partial support" in patients with heart failure with less-advanced disease may be used before the onset of irreversible myocardial damage and end-organ dysfunction. It has been speculated

Competing interest statement: Dr Dowling is the Medical Director of SCR Inc, Louisville, KY and medical consultant for CircuLite Inc, Saddle Brook, NJ, Abiomed Inc, Danvers, MA, and Evaheart Medical Inc, Pittsburgh, PA.

[a] MD/PhD Program, Department of Physiology and Biophysics, University of Louisville School of Medicine, Louisville, KY, USA
[b] Department of Surgery, University of Louisville, Louisville, KY, USA
* Corresponding author. 310 West Liberty Street, Suite 604, Louisville, KY 40202.
E-mail address: robddowling@gmail.com

Cardiol Clin 29 (2011) 559–582
doi:10.1016/j.ccl.2011.08.013
0733-8651/11/$ – see front matter © 2011 Elsevier Inc. All rights reserved.

that partial unloading of the failing left ventricle interrupts the progressive hemodynamic deterioration observed in heart failure[7] as well as increases functional capacity, improves quality of life, and promotes myocardial recovery. Although there are limited data to support this hypothesis, initial clinical results with partial-support devices are encouraging.[7,17,19,20]

Right ventricular failure remains a major concern after orthotopic heart transplantation or the implantation of an LVAD and accounts for half of early mortality with an LVAD.[21–23] As the number of patients with LVADs increases, the incidence of right ventricular failure will also increase. As such, novel right ventricular assist devices (RVADs) that are easy to place and remove are gaining attention for the treatment of right ventricular failure.

In parallel, the total artificial heart (TAH) has gained further acceptance as a therapy for patients with irreversible biventricular failure.[24] The success of current TAHs has prompted industry to reduce the size of approved TAHs to fit in a broader range of body sizes. More recently, concurrent implantation of 2 continuous-flow, full-support devices has emerged as a potential long-term therapy for patients with biventricular failure.[25] If proved safe and efficacious, therapy with dual, intracorporeal rotary pumps adds an additional treatment modality for end-stage, biventricular failure.

As mechanical circulatory support gains prevalence in the clinical management of cardiovascular disease, it is increasingly important to raise awareness of novel systems, the unique physiologic mechanisms by which each device functions, and implications for patient management. This article discusses state-of-the-art devices that are currently being developed or are in clinical trials. Devices are categorized as (1) full support, (2) less-invasive full support, (3) partial support: rotary pumps, (4) partial support: counterpulsation devices, (5) RVAD, and (6) TAH. Implantation strategy, mechanism of action, durability, efficacy, hemocompatibility, and quality of life during device support are considered. The feasibility of novel strategies for unloading the failing heart are examined.

STANDARD FULL-SUPPORT LVADs

In the past 2 decades, full-support LVADs have evolved into a standard therapy for patients with end-stage heart failure[26–28] as a bridge to cardiac transplantation,[29] as destination therapy,[29] or as a bridge to myocardial recovery.[30,31] In 2002, the milestone REMATCH (Randomized Evaluation of Mechanical Assistance for the Treatment of Congestive Heart Failure) trial showed clinical success with pulsatile LVADs as a long-term therapy for patients with end-stage heart failure.[27] Subsequently, the US Food and Drug Administration (FDA) approved use of the pulsatile HeartMate XVE as a destination therapy device in patients ineligible for cardiac transplantation.[32]

More recently, first-generation pulsatile LVADs that mimic native cardiac function have been replaced by rotary blood pumps that continuously unload the failing left ventricle.[33] In 2008 and 2010, the FDA approved the HeartMate II continuous-flow LVAD for patients as a bridge to transplant[34] and then as a destination therapy,[35] respectively. Compared with first-generation pulsatile devices, the HeartMate II and other second-generation continuous-flow devices are smaller, more reliable and durable, more energy efficient, less thrombogenic, and less surgically traumatic to implant. Importantly, superior clinical outcomes have been established with continuous-flow devices. With nearly 3000 patients logged, the Interagency Registry for Mechanically Assisted Circulatory Support (INTERMACS) documented a recent 1-year survival rate of 75%.[36]

However, better clinical outcomes are necessary before prolonged LVAD support is more widely accepted. For example, currently approved devices contain parts that wear out, such as polymeric valves and diaphragms or mechanical contact bearings. To counter this limitation and increase device durability, third-generation full-support devices include a bearingless, magnetically suspended impeller that does not wear with time or generate frictional heat.[6] Lack of pulsatile blood flow, excessive anticoagulation, device-induced coagulopathy, pump thrombosis, and morbidity related to driveline infections have also raised concerns. Consequently, continuous-flow pulsation algorithms are being developed to generate pulsatility,[37,38] textured interior surfaces have been revisited to minimize anticoagulation requirements and clotting,[39] and totally implantable systems with transcutaneous energy transfer (TET) technology are gaining attention.[40] As device companies incorporate these features into new systems, full-support LVAD therapy is likely to further increase in clinical success and prevalence. In the near future, the Thoratec HeartMate III, Cleveland Heart CorAide, and EVAHEART LVAS hold promise as novel, full-support LVADs.

HeartMate III

The HeartMate III (Thoratec Corporation, Pleasanton, CA) is a compact (69×30 mm; 535 g; 175 mL displacement), bearingless centrifugal-flow LVAD with a magnetically levitated impeller that is designed for long-term destination therapy.[4] Via median sternotomy, the flexible inflow cannula (**Fig. 1**A) is inserted in the left ventricular apex. The outflow graft is sewn end-to-side to the ascending aorta (see **Fig. 1**B). As blood is drawn into the device, the impeller imparts angular acceleration to the blood flow as it is delivered into the aorta. The patient wears an extracorporeal driver and electronics.

The HeartMate III includes several attractive features. The magnetically suspended bearing eliminates friction wear and may permit continuous support of up to 11 L/min for more than a decade.[4,41] At 4000 to 5000 rpm, the HeartMate III can generate 7 L/min of flow against a pump head pressure of 135 mm Hg while consuming less than 10 W of power. Control of the device is achieved with an autoresponsive algorithm based on motor parameters. As afterload and preload change, the device performance parameters are automatically adjusted to maintain the same flow.

Magnetic levitation permits precise control of the impeller. Radial suspension and rotation are actively controlled. Tilting and axial motion are passively controlled without power consumption. In the event of a device component failure, the electronics are designed with single fault-tolerant redundancy to ensure uninterrupted flow.[4] Similar to the Thoratec HeartMate II, a sensorless algorithm based on the relationship between power consumption, rotor speed, and electrical current estimates device flow.[42]

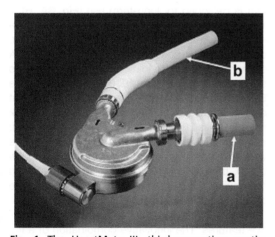

Fig. 1. The HeartMate III, third-generation continuous-flow centrifugal device, is shown with inflow cannula (a) and outflow graft (b). (*From* Farrar DJ, Bourque K, Dague CP, et al. Design features, developmental status, and experimental results with the HeartMate III centrifugal left ventricular assist system with a magnetically levitated rotor. ASAIO J 2007; 53:310–5; with permission.)

The driveline of the HeartMate III attaches to the device with a hermetically sealing quick connector. This modular approach separates cable reliability from pump reliability, which may permits an upgrade from a percutaneously powered system to a TET power source.[4] The current percutaneous version includes a belt-mounted driver and pair of batteries, which allow untethered mobility for up to 6 hours.[4] A tethered configuration provides uninterrupted power from a standard wall electrical socket to the device. The totally implantable version is currently being developed and is expected to minimize device-related infections and improve psychological and physical quality of life.

To minimize the potential for thromboembolism and to decrease anticoagulant pharmacotherapy, sintered titanium coats all blood-contacting surfaces except the smooth titanium impeller.[4] In the Thoratec HeartMate XVE, a textured surface successfully promoted in-growth of a fibrocellular, pseudoneointimal lining that lowered the risk of thromboembolic complications.[39] In these patients, daily aspirin alone provided sufficient anticoagulation. In addition, large gaps between the HeartMate III impeller and impeller housing provide channels outside the main blood flow path to wash internal device components.

An artificial pulse mode was developed to generate permanent or intermittent pulsatile blood flow.[37] In an acute ovine model with cardiectomy, by rapidly increasing and decreasing the rotational speed of the magnetically suspended impeller, a pulse pressure of up to 33 mm Hg was achieved.[37,43] The clinical relevance of pulsatility during mechanical circulatory support is unclear.[33] However, pulsatile blood flow is an important component of cardiovascular homeostasis that may have important implications for endothelial function, cardiac and arterial architecture and remodeling, end-organ perfusion, and weaning from a device. It remains to be determined whether induced pulsatility with an LVAD will improve long-term clinical outcomes.

Extensive preclinical testing of the HeartMate III is underway. Mock circulatory loop testing is ongoing with a goal of 80% reliability with 60% confidence at 5 years.[4] In a chronic bovine model that included a subset of animals studied according to a good laboratory practices (GLP) standard,[4] the HeartMate III generated flow of up to 11 L/min during 90-day experiments. Hemolysis and tissue heating did not occur. End organs were functionally normal and free of infarction.

Additional preclinical testing in an acute ovine model showed successful biventricular assist device (BiVAD) therapy after native cardiectomy with and without induced pulsation.[37,43] In a chronic bovine model, dual HeartMate III implantation successfully supported a calf for 20 days and established the feasibility of long-term continuous-flow BiVAD therapy.[44] The potential for dual intracorporeal support with native cardiectomy is significant and is discussed later in this article.

CorAide

The CorAide blood pump (Cleveland Heart Incorporated, Charlotte, NC) is a magnetically levitated, centrifugal continuous-flow LVAD.[14] The CorAide LVAD is implanted via median sternotomy with extracorporeal circulation. The inflow cannula resides within the left ventricular apex, and the outflow graft is anastomosed end-to-side to the aorta. The pump contains a cast-titanium volute housing (84 mL volume displacement, 293 g), a rotating magnetic ring with impeller veins, and a fluorinated ethylene-propylene (FEP)–coated titanium stator (**Fig. 2**, left). Plans are being made to replace the FEP-coated stator with BioMedFlex, a hard carbon coating.[45] The rotating ring spins around the stator post suspended in the axial direction by magnetic forces and in the radial direction by a thin layer of blood. This innovative blood-lubricated film bearing eliminates blood stagnation, mechanical wear and heat generation, and has shown significant tolerance to motion and mechanical impact.[46] A driveline is externalized to a portable electronics module powered through a standard wall socket or 2 nickel-metal hydride batteries, which may provide up to 6 hours of support.[47] The lightweight controller (1.35 kg) facilitates patient mobility.[14] At a flow of 5.5 L/min, the CorAide consumes approximately 6 W.[48]

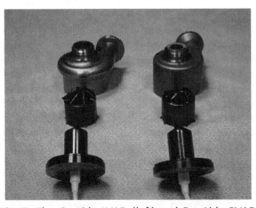

Fig. 2. The CorAide LVAD (*left*) and DexAide RVAD (*right*) are third generation continuous-flow devices. Internal components are shown. (*From* Saeed D, Ootaki Y, Ootaki C, et al. Acute in vivo evaluation of an implantable continuous flow biventricular assist system. ASAIO J 2008;54(1):20–4; with permission.)

Extensive preclinical testing of the CorAide LVAD has been performed in 53 animals for 30 or 90 days.[47–49] In 18 chronic animals, hemodynamics were stable, and there were no instances of bleeding, organ dysfunction, or mechanical failure.[49] Six implants have been successfully conducted without anticoagulation.[50]

In a European trial, an earlier version of the CorAide was implanted in 2 male patients with a follow-up of more than 6 months. Both patients had an uneventful postoperative course, and no thromboembolic events, hemolysis, infection, or mechanical failures occurred. In both patients, preoperative cardiac output increased from less than 3.25 L/min to 5.6 L/min, cardiac index doubled, and pulmonary capillary wedge pressure was reduced by half.[14] Both patients were anticoagulated because of atrial fibrillation. Despite excellent pump performance and biocompatibility, postexplant analysis showed delamination of the FEP coating. Subsequently, BioMedFlex has been introduced into the CorAide (and DexAide RVAD, described later) as a new journal-bearing material for cardiac assist devices. In chronic animal testing with this material, delamination was not observed, and biologic deposition did not occur.[45]

EVAHEART LVAS

The EVAHEART LVAS (EVAHEART Medical Incorporated, Pittsburgh, PA; Sun Medical Technology Research Corporation, Nagano, Japan) is a full-support centrifugal pump (55×76 mm, 420 g) that is designed for long-term use (**Fig. 3**A, B).[51] Through a median sternotomy, the inflow cannula is placed in the left ventricular apex, and the outflow graft is sewn to the ascending aorta. A sensorless, brushless, direct-current motor drives the impeller (40 mm) at 1900 to 2600 rpm. The EVAHEART LVAS was designed with a flat pressure-flow relationship that enables a peak flow of up to 20 L/min with a low-pressure head. Large inflow and outflow cannulas (16 mm), as well as the wide cross-sectional area of the pump, provide a low-resistance flow path within the device. A portable external driver powers the device (see **Fig. 3**A).

The EVAHEART LVAS contains several attractive features. The innovative combination of a flat pressure-flow relationship and a wide flow pathway generates a significant increase in flow during native ventricular systole that results in a wide pulse pressure. To improve hemocompatibility, the blood-contacting surfaces are coated with 2-methylacryloyloxyethyl phosphorylcholine (MPC), an antithrombogenic organic zwitterion

A   **B**

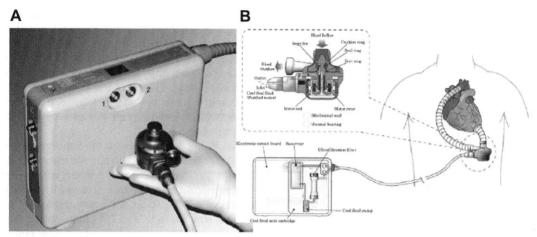

Fig. 3. The EVAHEART LVAS is a full-support centrifugal pump. (*A*) The device and the control unit. (*B*) Device design and implant position. (*From* Takatani S, Matsuda H, Hanatani A, et al. Mechanical circulatory support devices (MCSD) in Japan: current status and future directions. J Artif Organs 2005;8(1):13–27; with permission.)

found on the surface of erythrocytes.[52,53] A low-temperature mechanical seal fuses the shaft.[54] Recirculated sterile water continuously flushes the inner faces of the seal to improve convective heat transfer and prevent heat denaturation of serum proteins. An extended durability of up to 10 years of support is expected.

In an acute bovine model, during exercise the EVAHEART LVAS automatically increased pump flow without a change in revolutions per minute.[55] At a constant pump speed, exercise increased systolic pump flow by a factor of 3 and indicated a sensitive responsiveness to preload and changing heart rate during increased total-body metabolic demands.

In a chronic bovine model, through a left thoracotomy, the EVAHEART LVAS successfully supported calves for 3 to 7 months.[51] At 3 to 5 L/min, the pump consumed 8 to 10 W. During treadmill exercise, pump flow exceeded 10 L/min. No hemolysis occurred, and 6 of 10 animals survived to elective termination. At necropsy, there was no evidence of infection or pump thrombus on the blood-contacting surfaces of the inflow cannula, outflow graft, or pump. A few small renal infarcts were noted.[51,53] In additional chronic calves, MPC coating of blood-contacting surfaces significantly reduced activated platelets compared with a diamondlike carbon coating.[53] In this study, 3 animals were successfully supported without postoperative anticoagulation.

In May 2005, a clinical trial was initiated at 4 centers in Japan.[18] An initial report of 2 patients describes functional class improvements from New York Heart Association (NYHA) class IV to class I without adverse events at 603 and 543 days of support.[56] Patients showed an aortic pulse pressure of 20 to 30 mm Hg. In December 2010, the Japanese Pharmaceutical and Medical Device Agency approved the EVAHEART LVAS for bridge to transplantation. A multicenter trial is currently underway in the United States with an Investigational Device Exemption (IDE). This trial may help to determine whether the potential advantages of the device (preserved pulse pressure, antithrombogenic coating, extended durability) may translate into improved, long-term patient outcomes.

LESS-INVASIVE FULL-SUPPORT DEVICES

If combined, the benefits of a full-support device implanted with a minimally invasive surgical approach may expand the potential patient population for LVAD therapy. As LVADs are miniaturized, minimally invasive implantation may increase acceptance by patients and physicians who are more likely to refer patients for less-invasive surgical therapies.[57] As a result, earlier intervention in less-sick patients may increase the public-health impact of mechanical circulatory support. Novel surgical approaches may include limited thoracotomy, subxiphoid access, thoracic keyhole access, placement of surface devices, or percutaneous implantation.

Furthermore, these operative approaches often do not require cardiopulmonary bypass.[58] As a result, less postoperative coagulopathy may reduce postoperative bleeding and blood transfusions that play a role in right ventricular dysfunction and infection with LVADs.[59] In the near future, the HeartWare MVAD holds promise as a small, full-support rotary pump with multiple configurations that may be implanted without a sternotomy or extracorporeal circulation.

Miniature Ventricular Assist Device

The miniature ventricular assist device (MVAD; HeartWare Incorporated, Miami Lakes, FL) platform technology is based on a small (15 mL displacement), bearingless, axial-flow LVAD.[5] Within a cylindrical titanium housing, an electromagnetic motor stator powers a magnetically levitated, wide-blade impeller with a large surface area to produce hydrodynamic thrust bearings. Small gaps minimize the distance between magnetic poles and the stator and provide impeller stability. The combination of hydrodynamic thrust bearings and an axial–suspended impeller eliminate upstream and downstream support structures. This innovative design produces a platform for multiple device configurations that may be implanted through less-invasive surgical approaches but still provide full-support therapy. At 12,000 to 20,000 rpm, the MVAD generates up to 8 L/min of flow. Hydrodynamic thrust bearings that are larger than the main blood flow paths passively suspend the rotor. The patient wears an extracorporeal power source and electronics.

The small housing is one-third the size of HeartWare's predicate HVAD (**Fig. 4**A #3) and can be manufactured in 3 configurations that are currently being investigated.[60] Two configurations use a transapical approach, and a third configuration uses a transmitral approach. The first transapical MVAD configuration is implanted with a left thoracotomy or median sternotomy. The cylindrical inflow/pump housing of the device is implanted through the left ventricular apex (see **Fig. 4**A #2, B), and the base of the device resides within the pericardium. A 10-mm double-woven outflow graft angled at 90° from the base of the device is anastomosed end-to-side to the descending aorta.

A second, transapical MVAD configuration is implanted with a subxiphoid approach.[60] After entering the pericardium through a small incision below the xiphoid process, the device is inserted through the left ventricular apex to reside within the left ventricular chamber (see **Fig. 4**A #4, C). The inflow of the device unloads up to 8 L/min of blood volume from within the left ventricle through an outflow cannula that is permanently positioned across the aortic valve (see **Fig. 4**C). This novel approach places a continuous-flow LVAD in series (rather than in parallel) with the circulation, obviates an outflow graft anastomosis, and dramatically reduces the invasiveness and length of the implantation procedure. Intraventricular placement may also eliminate device pocket infections.[5] The long-term effects on the aortic valve and the incidence of thromboembolism remain to be defined.

The transmitral MVAD configuration is implanted through a small, right-sided thoracotomy (see **Fig. 4**A #1, D). A flexible inflow cannula is implanted in the left atrium through Waterson's groove between the right superior and inferior pulmonary veins. The tip of the inflow cannula is positioned across the mitral valve into the left ventricle. The outflow graft is sewn to the ascending aorta.

In a chronic bovine model, the first transapical MVAD configuration was implanted successfully for 30 days. Measurement of cardiac output with the thermodilution technique showed that pump speeds of 19,500 to 21,3000 rpm generated an average flow of 4.25 ($\pm$ 0.75) L/min, which was approximately 80% of cardiac output. After euthanasia, the explanted device was free of thrombus, no thermal damage was present, and end organs were free of infarction.[5] Preclinical testing of the other 2 MVAD configurations is currently underway.

PARTIAL-SUPPORT DEVICES: ROTARY PUMPS

If a patient on a cardiac transplant waiting list is worsening and an appropriate organ is not available, a full-support LVAD may be the only option for survival. However, many patients with heart failure are not ill enough to warrant or have contraindications to placement of a full-support LVAD. In these patients, the notion of combining the benefits of partial support with a minimally invasive and short operation without cardiopulmonary bypass may be feasible. A recent National Heart, Lung, and Blood Institute (NHLBI) mission statement included the pursuit of long-term hemodynamic support with minimally invasive surgery to provide moderate levels of mechanical assistance earlier in the progression of heart failure (NHLBI, Clinical Use of Ventricular Assist Devices Working Group, March 27–28, 2008 Crystal City, VA).[61] The long-term benefits of chronic, partial unloading of the failing left ventricle are unknown but may soon be characterized by present clinical trials.[7] Significant clinical benefit has been predicted[62] and may decrease the number of patients who require a transplant.

For example, a large gap in available therapies exists for patients in NYHA class III who have not responded to biventricular pacing. If these patients are transplant ineligible or have not met hemodynamic and clinical criteria to justify the risks and comorbidities of sternotomy and a full-support LVAD, limited options exist. In these patients, partial support with a less-invasive device is an attractive option. If partial support is administered early enough, favorable reverse

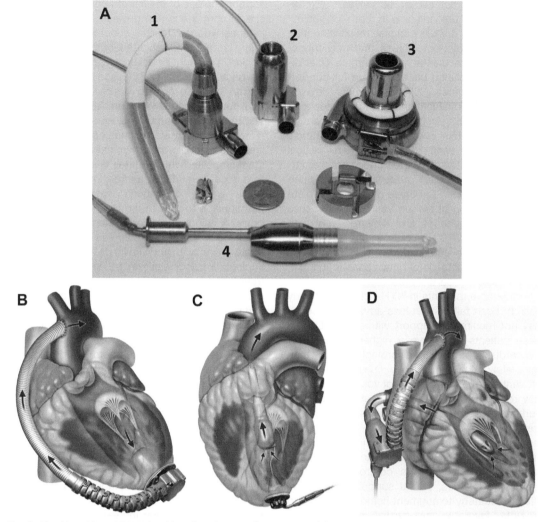

Fig. 4. The HeartWare HVAD (*A* #3) and various configurations of the HeartWare MVAD in development (*A* #1, 2, 4) are shown. The first transapical MVAD configuration is implanted through the left ventricular apex (*A* #2, *B*) with the outflow graft sewn to the descending aorta. The second, transapical MVAD configuration is implanted with a subxiphoid approach (*A* #4, *C*). The transmitral MVAD configuration is implanted through a small, right-sided thoracotomy (*A* #1, *D*). (*Courtesy of* HeartWare Inc (Miami Lakes, FL); with permission. *Courtesy of* Daniel Tamez.)

myocardial remodeling may occur and permit explantation of the device.[63] This hypothesis has not been rigorously tested but is conceptually appealing.

Indeed mounting evidence suggests that full support of the failing left ventricle with an LVAD can promote reverse myocardial remodeling and LVAD explantation in select patients.[30,31] In these instances, functional recovery has been accompanied by favorable changes at the molecular, histologic, and functional levels.[64,65] However, strategies to promote myocardial recovery with a full-support LVAD have shown limited success.

Furthermore, with time, maximum volume unloading of the left ventricle may be detrimental to the cardiovascular system. As the level of full-support therapy increases, variation in end-systolic and end-diastolic volumes diminishes and eliminates the native workload of the heart.[33] As a result, myocyte atrophy[66,67] and ventricular stiffening[68] may occur and preclude myocardial recovery. Simultaneously, complete volume unloading of the heart decreases peak systolic left ventricular pressures to the point at which the aortic valve remains chronically closed and may result in fused valve leaflets, acquired aortic stenosis, or total occlusive thrombosis of prosthetic aortic valves.[69] Excessive ventricular unloading with both pulsatile[70] and continuous[71] LVADs can also result in suction events and ventricular collapse that may trigger episodes of ventricular tachyarrhythmias. Of additional concern, during therapy with a full-support LVAD, approximately 30% of patients develop right ventricular dysfunction[22] with an associated mortality of 43%.[23] An abrupt increase in cardiac output can acutely overload the right ventricle and cause right ventricular failure. Early clinical data suggest that partial support does not dramatically increase cardiac output and right-sided overload is unlikely.[7] For these reasons, complete volume unloading of the left ventricle may cause adverse consequences and limit recovery with a full-support LVAD. In contrast, partial support may avoid these complications but still provide adequate augmentation of native cardiac function and promote myocardial recovery.

Furthermore, patients in NYHA class III or early class IV heart failure with less-advanced disease may not require full support with an LVAD, and these patients may have a higher likelihood of myocardial recovery.[62] Accordingly, rather than completely unloading blood volume from the failing left ventricle, earlier and partial volume unloading may reduce, but not eliminate, native ventricular workload, preserve myocardial structure, and prevent myocardial atrophy and stiffening. By reducing ventricular workload and augmenting myocardial blood flow while still allowing the heart to fill and empty within a controlled range of ventricular volumes, partial support may be an effective strategy to augment hemodynamics and promote favorable myocardial remodeling in hearts with less disease. With this goal in mind, the CircuLite Synergy pocket micropump was designed. Recent clinical results are encouraging.

CircuLite Synergy Pocket Micropump

The CircuLite Synergy pocket micropump (CircuLite Incorporated, Saddle Brook, NJ, USA) is a small continuous-flow device the size of an AA battery (**Fig. 5A**, 49 mm, outer diameter 14 mm, 25 g).[19] The CircuLite LVAD is implanted via a right-sided mini-thoracotomy without extracorporeal circulation. Via modified Seldinger technique, the inflow cannula is implanted between the right superior and inferior pulmonary veins and positioned in the left atrium. Left atrial versus left ventricular cannulation with a continuous-flow LVAD provides similar flow rates, and left ventricular volumes and energetic parameters decrease with increasing pump speed irrespective of cannulation site.[72] These data and the clinical experience described later

support the use of the left atrium as a cannulation site for continuous-flow devices. The outflow graft is anastomosed to the subclavian artery. The pump is implanted subcutaneously in a pacemaker pocket in the right infraclavicular groove anterior to the pectoralis major muscle (see **Fig. 5B–D**).

The CircuLite Synergy Pump is designed to continuously, partially unload 2.5 to 3.0 L/min of blood from the left atrium into the subclavian artery. A brushless, microelectric motor powers a magnetically stabilized, hydrodynamically levitated single-stage impeller, which rotates at 20,000 to 28,000 rpm. Axial, centrifugal, and orthogonal blood flow paths ensure continuous washing of internal components to reduce the risk of impeller thrombosis. A nitinol-reinforced silicone inflow cannula (length 20.5 cm, inner diameter 6 mm) includes a Dacron cuff with titanium tip designed to facilitate implantation and healing in the left atrium. A polytetrafluoroethylene (PTFE) outflow cannula (inner diameter 8 mm) is trimmed to the appropriate length during the implantation procedure. A percutaneous lead exits the body from the right upper quadrant and connects to a controller and dual battery pack (1.5 kg), which permit approximately 16 to 18 hours of untethered mobility.[73]

Original theoretic work suggested that continuous, partial support of a failing ventricle may increase cardiac output and lower ventricular filling pressures.[62] The greatest hemodynamic benefits were predicted for less-dilated and less-dysfunctional hearts. Computer simulations were validated in an acute bovine model of cardiac dysfunction in which continuous partial support at a rate of 3 L/min decreased left atrial pressure by 6 to 7 mm Hg and increased cardiac output by greater than 1 L/min.[62] Ongoing bench testing has suggested long-term durability. Nine Synergy pumps that have run in a mock circulatory loop for 30 months have not shown mechanical wear at the pivot bearing.[7]

In an ongoing multicenter European clinical trial,[7] ionotrope-independent ambulatory patients on the transplant list with NYHA class IIIB or IVA heart failure and preserved end-organ function showed hemodynamic improvements in a 3-month follow-up,[7,19,73] with an ongoing maximum support duration of 8 months. Partial hemodynamic recovery included significant increases in cardiac index from 2.0 ± 0.4 to 2.8 ± 0.6 L/min/m^2, an increase in mean arterial pressure from 67 ± 8 to 80 ± 9 mm Hg, and a reduction in pulmonary capillary wedge pressure from 30 ± 5 to 18 ± 5 mm Hg.[19] N-terminal fragment probrain natriuretic peptide was significantly reduced from 6452 ± 5470 to 3209 ± 2379 pg/mL,[73] and suggested decreased myocyte mechanical stress.

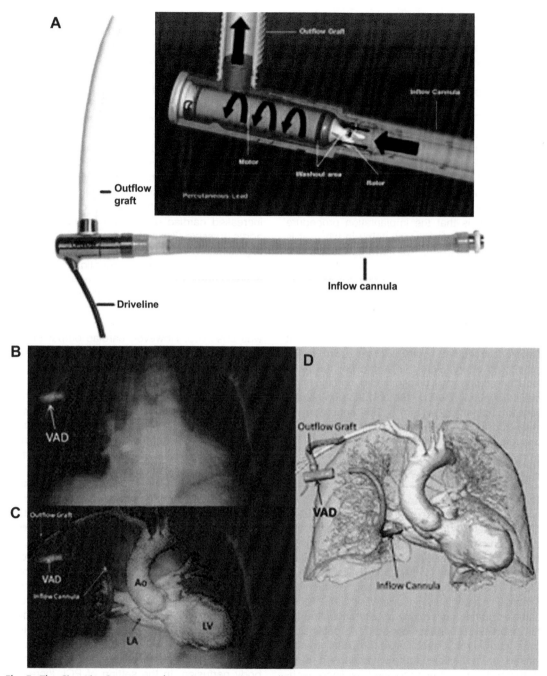

Fig. 5. The CirculLite Synergy pocket micropump is a small, partial-support LVAD (*A*). Radiograph and computed tomography scans show the position of pump in vivo (*B–D*). Ao, aorta; LA, left atrium; LV, left ventricle; SA, subclavian artery; VAD, ventricular assist device. (*From* (*A*) Meyns BP, Simon A, Klotz S, et al. Clinical benefits of partial circulatory support in New York Heart Association class IIIB and early class IV patients. Eur J Cardiothorac Surg 2011;39(5):693–8; with permission; and (*B–D*) Meyns B, Ector J, Rega F, et al. First human use of partial left ventricular heart support with the Circulite Synergy Micropump as a bridge to cardiac transplantation. Eur Heart J 2008;29(20):2582; with permission.)

As predicted, right heart failure was not a clinical challenge with the CircuLite pump. During support, the acute increase in cardiac output ranged from 1.0 to 1.5 L/min and did not overload the right ventricle.[7] However, this clinical trial did have adverse events. During the first 30 days of support, serious adverse events that included bleeding, infection, stroke, pump thrombosis, and pump exchange occurred at approximately half the rate reported for the HeartMate II.[7]

After 30 days of support pump thrombosis and pump exchange accounted for more than one-third of the adverse events reported.[7] As a result, modifications were made that included an increased size of the washout channels and redesign of the impeller and control algorithms, which have reduced the rate of pump thrombosis.[73] Notwithstanding, a great advantage is that the Synergy pump may be easily and rapidly exchanged through the original infraclavicular incision without entering the chest.

An additional and unique advantage of the CircuLite pump is that the implantation procedure involves a right-sided thoracotomy in which it is unlikely that adhesions will form in the anterior mediastinum and complicate median sternotomy if heart transplantation is indicated. A future design that obviates entrance into the thorax may include a percutaneous inflow graft placed through the subclavian vein and advanced through the interatrial septum into the left atrium. As with the current design, the outflow graft will be sewn to the subclavian artery. With this approach, the need for a thoracotomy will be eliminated, and the infraclavicular incision will be the only incision necessary to implant the system.[73] This approach will likely further increase acceptance by patients and referring physicians.

Reitan Catheter Pump

The Reitan catheter pump (CardioBridge, Hechingen, Germany) is a novel, intra-aortic, propeller-based catheter pump (**Fig. 6**A).[10] In patients with cardiogenic shock or in patients undergoing high-risk percutaneous coronary intervention (PCI) in whom an intra-aortic balloon pump (IABP) is contraindicated because of tachyarrhythmia or aortic valve incompetence, the Reitan catheter pump may provide an alterative strategy for short-term cardiac support. A collapsible cage surrounds a retractable propeller that is loaded on a flexible catheter (collapsed outer diameter 4.6 mm). Via a modified Seldinger technique, the catheter is introduced percutaneously into the high ascending aorta (see **Fig. 6**B, C). In vivo, the cage is deployed and the propeller blades are extended and rapidly rotated. With rotational speeds of 10,000 to 14,000 rpm, a pressure gradient of up to 25 mm Hg is produced across the propeller, which unloads the left ventricle by reducing pressure in the aortic arch proximal to the pump. Distal to the pump, augmented blood pressure increases perfusion of the abdominal organs and lower half of the

body. The proximal end of the catheter is connected to an external drive unit and user console.

The hydraulic properties of the Reitan catheter pump have been evaluated in mock circulatory loops.[74] The generated pressure reduction was related to the size of the mock aorta. The aortic diameter influenced the pressure gradient that developed across the propeller. In larger aortas, a deceased pressure gradient was likely because of backflow around the tips of the rotating propeller blades. Clinically, this finding suggests that the Reitan catheter pump may be most effective in patients with smaller aortas.

In normal pigs, the Reitan catheter pump increased cardiac output and reduced proximal aortic pressure.[75] In a bovine model of acute mitral regurgitation, the Reitan catheter pump caused significant rpm-dependent reductions in mean ascending aortic pressure that reached −10 mm Hg and in left ventricular peak systolic pressure, an indirect index of myocardial metabolic demand. A significant increase in abdominal aortic pressure was observed. However, cardiac output did not improve, and negative pressure in the ascending aorta decreased carotid artery flow and mean diastolic coronary artery flow (net coronary blood flow was unaffected because of an increased contribution in systolic coronary flow).[76] Similarly, in a bovine model of pharmacologically induced acute heart failure, the Reitan catheter pump significantly decreased left ventricular systolic pressure by approximately 20 mm Hg and left atrial pressure by 5 mm Hg, and increased femoral pressure by 19 mm Hg. A 15% reduction in carotid artery blood flow was observed. Coronary artery, renal, and femoral blood flow were unchanged.[77]

In a randomized clinical trial in 10 patients, the Reitan catheter pump safely provided cardiac support during PCI.[10] No deaths or strokes occurred. No significant hemolysis occurred, and platelet function was unchanged. At rotational speeds of 10,500 rpm, an aortic pressure gradient of approximately 10 mm Hg was maintained across the pump. An improvement in renal function suggested increased abdominal and lower body perfusion. In the setting of PCI, increased renal perfusion may protect against contrast nephropathy. However, this hypothesis remains to be tested with this device.

Procyon Circulatory Assist Device

The Procyon circulatory assist device (CAD; Procyon Incorporated, Houston, TX) is a catheter-deployed intra-aortic, continuous-flow LVAD designed for long-term partial circulatory support. The Procyon CAD consists of a miniature rotary

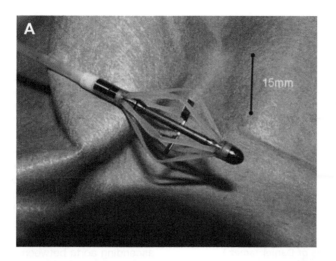

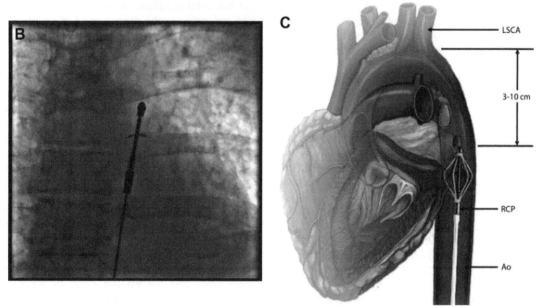

Fig. 6. The Reitan catheter pump (RCP) shown ex vivo (*A*), in vivo (*B*), and in a schematic diagram (*C*). LSCA, left subclavian artery. (*From* Smith EJ, Reitan O, Keeble T, et al. A first-in-man study of the Reitan catheter pump for circulatory support in patients undergoing high-risk percutaneous coronary intervention. Catheter Cardiovasc Interv 2009;73(7):859–65; with permission.)

pump caged within a catheter-based nitinol strut system (**Fig. 7**A, deployed; B, collapsed). Via a percutaneous approach, the catheter-based pump is advanced and permanently deployed in the descending aorta. As with the Reitan catheter pump, the Procyon CAD unloads the left ventricle by decreasing proximal aortic resistance while providing distal aortic flow augmentation.

In a mock circulatory loop, the Procyon CAD improved mean arterial pressure by 5%, cardiac output by 6%, and decreased left ventricular external work by 15%. In an acute ovine model of pharmacologically induced heart failure, the

Procyon CAD moderately increased dP/dt and increased cardiac output from 3.5 to 4.6 L/min (unpublished results, Reynolds Delgado, MD, 2011).

PARTIAL-SUPPORT DEVICES: COUNTERPULSATION DEVICES

Counterpulsation with an IABP is the most common mechanical circulatory support strategy for a wide variety of cardiovascular disorders. Although IABP implantation does not require major surgery, during IABP support the patient must

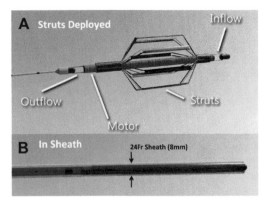

Fig. 7. The Procyon circulatory assist device is shown with struts deployed (*A*) and collapsed before deployment (*B*). (*Courtesy of* HeartWare Inc (Miami Lakes, FL); with permission. *Courtesy of* Daniel Tamez.)

remain supine and is thereby immobilized and susceptible to numerous complications. Biocompatibility issues typically limit IABP therapy to short durations of hours to days. When IABP therapy is used for prolonged periods of greater than 20 days, the frequency of vascular complications, bleeding, and infection is high and is associated with increased mortality.[78,79]

Nevertheless, decades of widespread success with the IABP for short-term indications have generated interest in long-term counterpulsation strategies. Multiple surgical approaches (aortomyoplasty,[80] skeletal muscle ventricle[81]), and invasive devices (Paraaortic counterpulsation device,[82] CardioVAD[17]) were intended to supplement cardiac function for long-term therapy. However, these approaches required sternotomy or thoracotomy.

In patients with severe hemodynamic impairment, chronic counterpulsation does not provide the same degree of support as an LVAD and is not a suitable option. However, less-invasive chronic counterpulsation may be a practical partial-support strategy to expand treatment options and improve quality of life in a large cohort of patients with less advanced heart failure.

As discussed previously, early partial support may promote reverse myocardial remodeling. The objectives of counterpulsation are to (1) generate an ancillary pressure pulse during native ventricular diastole to augment diastolic pressure and increase coronary and systemic blood flow (increase supply), and (2) decrease aortic pressure during native ventricular systole to reduce vascular afterload and ventricular work (decrease demand). Both of these mechanisms favorably affect myocardial mechanoenergetics. Consequently, long-term counterpulsation may promote myocardial recovery by rebalancing the myocardial oxygen supply/demand relationship. However, chronic ambulatory counterpulsation has not been rigorously evaluated, and this hypothesis remains to be tested. With this goal in mind, 2 novel devices, the Sunshine Heart C-Pulse and the SCR Symphony device have been developed for less-invasive, long-term counterpulsation.

C-Pulse

The C-Pulse (Sunshine Heart Incorporated, Tustin, CA, USA) is an implantable, extra-aortic counterpulsation device.[9] Via median sternotomy or right anterior thoracotomy without cardiopulmonary bypass, a polyester-coated polyurethane balloon cuff is installed circumferentially around the ascending aorta between the sinotubular junction and the brachiocephalic artery. Cuffs accommodate ascending aortic diameters of 28 to 40 mm. A minimum length of 70 mm of aorta is needed. A bipolar epicardial electrocardiographic lead (Capsure Epi 65 cm, Medtronic Incorporated, Stillwater, MN, USA) is attached to the right ventricular outflow tract to trigger the device. A driveline is passed from the thorax subcutaneously through the abdominal wall. At the percutaneous exit site, a connector fastens the driveline to a portable pneumatic driver (**Fig. 8**A).

The C-Pulse functions by classic counterpulsation in series with the cardiovascular system. Just after closure of the aortic valve during native diastole, the balloon cuff inflates and compresses the ascending aortic wall. The thumbprint deflection of the outer curvature of the aorta displaces 20 to 30 mL of aortic root blood volume toward the heart to increase diastolic coronary artery blood flow, and toward the body to augment end-organ perfusion (see **Fig. 8**B). The R-wave on the electrocardiogram triggers the balloon cuff to deflate. As a result, central aortic end-diastolic blood pressure decreases and reduces the metabolic demands of the heart necessary to eject through the aortic valve (see **Fig. 8**C).

In an acute porcine model, extra-aortic balloon counterpulsation with a 7-mL balloon cuff outperformed a 25-mL IABP in diastolic coronary blood flow augmentation and performed comparably in diastolic pressure augmentation, afterload reduction, and augmentation of cardiac output.[83] Histopathologic changes were not observed in the ascending aortic tunica intima or tunica media. However, mild hemorrhagic inflammatory changes were observed in the tunica adventitia.

A short-term intraoperative safety study was performed in 6 patients with normal ventricular function undergoing off-pump, first-time coronary artery bypass grafting. During C-Pulse support,

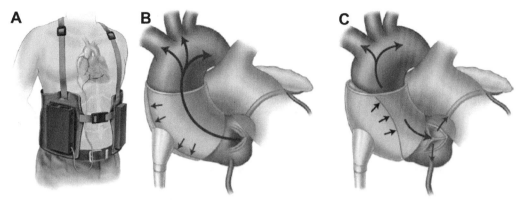

Fig. 8. The C-Pulse implantable, extra-aortic counterpulsation device with portable driver (*A*), in position around the aorta with balloon deflated (*B*) and inflated (*C*). (*From* Sales, VL, McCarthy PM. Understanding the C-pulse device and its potential to treat heart failure. Curr Heart Fail Rep 2010;7:27–34; with permission; and Davies AN, Peters WS, Su T, et al. Extra-ascending aortic versus intra-descending aortic balloon counterpulsation-effect on coronary artery blood flow. Heart Lung Circ 2005;14(3):178–86; with permission.)

transesophageal echocardiography showed a 31% reduction in left ventricular wall stress, a 16% reduction in left ventricular end-systolic area, and a 13% increase in fractional area change. Diastolic coronary blood flow increased by 67%.[84]

More recently, a prospective multicenter feasibility trial was initiated in the United States to evaluate the safety and efficacy of the C-Pulse in 20 patients with NYHA class III and IV heart failure. Initial success was reported.[20,85] All patients improved by at least 1 NYHA class. In 3 patients, right heart catheterization at 1 month showed an improvement in cardiac index and reduction in pulmonary artery pressures. Infection complicated device therapy in 60% of patients.[20] Aortic tissue retrieved at autopsy showed macroscopically normal aortic walls with an intact tunica intima and tunica media. Arterial remodeling was observed in some patients and included thickening of the adventitia, foreign-body response, neutrophilic infiltrate, and/or necrotic adventitia.

Perhaps the best feature of the C-Pulse is the absence of blood contact. As a result, anticoagulation is unnecessary. In addition, the device may be turned off safely at any point during support, which has been well received by patients, who have reported feeling less encumbered. Better mobility may translate into improved ability to perform activates of daily living, less device-related stress, and improved quality-of-life scores (personal communication, Sanjeev Aggarwal, MD, 2011). The limited operative approach and no postoperative anticoagulation may favorably affect patient outcomes by decreasing the incidence of thromboembolism, hemorrhage, and device-related coagulopathy.

The C-Pulse is contraindicated in patients with aortic regurgitation, severe disease of the ascending aorta, or patent aortocoronary bypass grafts. The long-term histopathologic effects to the aortic root and surrounding tissues have not been determined. In addition, the ease with which the device may be removed if operative therapies are needed (such as heart transplantation or full-support LVAD implantation) has not been reported. In the event of myocardial recovery, it may be possible to sever the driveline and leave the C-Pulse in situ to avoid a repeat, invasive procedure.

Symphony Counterpulsation Device

The Symphony counterpulsation device (SCR Incorporated, Louisville, KY, USA) is a peripheral counterpulsation device designed to deliver long-term, partial support without entering the thorax. In a simple surgical procedure, a valveless inflow/outflow cannula is anastomosed to the subclavian artery and attached to a pump with a 32-mL stroke volume (**Fig. 9**A). The pump is placed above the pectoralis major muscle in a subcutaneous pocket, similarly to a pacemaker (see **Fig. 9**B). To minimize complications associated with blood stasis and thrombosis, a constant but shifting vortex within the reservoir continuously washes the inside of the device. A percutaneous driveline exits in the right upper quadrant and attaches to a lightweight, portable pneumatic driver (20 × 10 × 10 cm, 1.5 kg) that is triggered by the patient's electrocardiogram.

The Symphony functions by counterpulsation with a peripheral capacitance chamber. Blood is removed from the circulation into the pump during

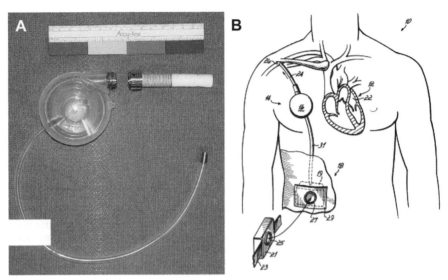

Fig. 9. The Symphony counterpulsation device is shown ex vivo (*A*) and in a schematic diagram (*B*). (*From* Bartoli CR, Wilson GC, Giridharan GA, et al. A novel subcutaneous counterpulsation device: acute hemodynamic efficacy during pharmacologically induced hypertension, hypotension, and heart failure. Artif Organs 2010;34(7):537–45; with permission.)

systole and returned to the circulation during diastole. As with standard counterpulsation devices that use volume displacement (rather than volume removal), the Symphony device results in afterload reduction during systole and coronary and systemic flow augmentation during diastole.[8] By these mechanisms, the Symphony improves the myocardial oxygen supply/demand ratio.[8]

Although the Symphony operates similarly to an IABP, the delivery of support is fundamentally different.[86,87] The surgical configuration does not influence the internal impedance of the aorta, and device filling and ejection are less dependent on timing than an IABP. With an IABP, inflation occurs immediately after aortic valve closure, and deflation must begin before the end of ventricular diastole to ensure that the balloon deflates and aortic resistance is low.[88] In contrast, the peripheral location of the Symphony may permit modest tradeoffs between improved coronary flow and left ventricular workload reduction.[86,87] Consequently, subtle variations in the delivery of support may have important implications for incremental patient management on an individualized basis. For example, ejection of the Symphony may be delayed until after isovolumetric relaxation when the coronary resistance is lowest, which may result in a modest additional increase in coronary artery flow compared with an IABP.[86,87] If filled before the beginning of ventricular systole, before the aortic valve opens, a large decrease in left ventricular ejection pressure translates into a larger reduction in ventricular work. Alternatively, filling

later during systole may result in less afterload reduction and may permit gradual reloading of the heart. Therefore, after an initial period of maximal counterpulsation therapy, left ventricular workload may be gradually increased to strengthen the myocardium and facilitate weaning of the device. If explantation is indicated, the Symphony may be surgically removed without entrance into the thorax.

The feasibility of effective counterpulsation via peripheral volume displacement with the Symphony has been validated in silico[86] and has been shown in vitro in a mock circulatory loop.[86,87] Efficacy has been confirmed in an acute bovine model.[8,87,89,90] These studies suggest that hemodynamic benefits with the Symphony are comparable with, or better than, an IABP in normal animals[87] and in animals with acute heart failure,[8] hypotension,[8] hypertension,[8] and chronic heart failure.[90] In preparation for clinical trials, long-term implants under GLP standards have been performed.

The implantation, operation, and management of an LVAD are cost-prohibitive for many health care systems, including China and India. As a result, the use of mechanical circulatory support in these markets is limited.[91] The Symphony device has a low manufacturing cost and can be implanted (and explanted) with a limited operative approach without extracorporeal circulation. Therefore, the Symphony may be a desirable alternative to the more invasive, expensive, and complex LVAD systems and may expand the use of mechanical circulatory support devices to these underserved markets.

RVADs

Right ventricular failure is a serious complication with a high mortality. Approximately 50% of all morbidity and 20% of early mortality after orthotopic heart transplantation relate to right ventricular failure.[21] Similarly, the acute increase in left ventricular output and septal shift with an LVAD produce right ventricular dysfunction in 30% of patients[22] with an associated mortality of 43%.[23] Although most patients recover with ionotropes and pulmonary vasodilators, right ventricular dysfunction remains a clinical challenge.

Few recent reports of next-generation implantable RVADs exist. The clinically approved Jarvik 2000 Flow Maker has been used off-label for right ventricular support.[92] Also in 2004, the pneumatically driven Thoratec implantable ventricular assist device (IVAD) was approved by the FDA for use as an implantable RVAD.[93] However, the large IVAD is not ideal for patient mobility outside the hospital setting. Anatomic compatibility of an RVAD with a preexisting LVAD is an additional and important consideration because of space constraints if an LVAD is present and because implantation of an isolated RVAD is rare.[94] Consequently, a small, next-generation implantable RVAD is still needed. The recent success of novel LVAD systems has bolstered interest in the development of next-generation RVAD systems.

DexAide

The DexAide Blood Pump (Cleveland Heart, Charlotte, NC) is a magnetically levitated, centrifugal pump[95] designed in parallel with the CorAide LVAD.[14] The DexAide contains a cast-titanium volute housing (44 × 48 mm, 69 mL volume displacement, 280 g), a rotating magnetic ring with impeller veins, and a zirconia (zirconium oxide) ceramic stator (see **Fig. 2**, right).[96] The rotating assembly spins around the stator post suspended in the axial direction by magnetic forces and in the radial direction by a blood-lubricated film.[97] Various inflow cannula designs and surgical implantation sites were rigorously tested for biocompatibility.[98] An open-ended titanium inflow cannula with 2 side openings positioned through the diaphragmatic surface of the right ventricle resulted in the least tissue deposition. The outflow cannula is anastomosed end-to-side to the trunk of the pulmonary artery. A driveline is externalized to a portable electronics module powered through a standard wall socket or 2 nickel-metal hydride batteries, which may

provide up to 12 hours of support.[96] Currently, Cleveland Heart is seeking an FDA IDE for the DexAide RVAD.[13]

In mock circulatory loops at 2450 rpm, the DexAide generated 4 L/min of flow and 40 mm Hg of pressure while consuming 3 W.[97] An 18-month in vitro endurance test has been completed.[13] In an acute bovine model, pump flow correlated with pump speed during high pulmonary arterial pressures but was limited during low-volume conditions. A right atrial pressure of at least 5 mm Hg was necessary to maintain sufficient pump flow.

In a chronic bovine model, an early version of the DexAide with a cast-titanium stator provided approximately 5 L/min of blood flow and consumed 3 W during 14-day to 90-day studies.[95,98] Subsequent in vitro[96] and 14-day to 91-day experiments[99] showed that the new zirconia ceramic stator reduced power consumption by 20% with similar hemodynamic performance to the original cast-titanium stator. No biologic deposition was observed on the new stator, which suggested that zirconia ceramic may be a useful material in the journal bearings of novel LVADs. In these experiments, a fixed-flow mode was successfully introduced to maintain target flow while preventing right ventricular suction events.[100]

Human-fit studies have been performed to simulate implantation of the DexAide in a patient with a preexisting HeartMate I or II, CorAide LVAD, or Novacor LVAD.[95,101,102] Findings indicated that implantation of the DexAide in the preperitoneal space interfered with the outflow conduit of the LVAD. As an alternative, implantation of the DexAide RVAD in the right chest cavity fit well with each LVAD.

The Cleveland Heart DexAide RVAD and CorAide LVAD have been developed in parallel for use as a continuous-flow BiVAD system.[103] The potential for dual intracorporeal support with small continuous-flow devices is significant and is discussed later in this review.

Impella Recover RD

The Impella Recover RD (Abiomed, Inc, Danvers, MA, USA) is an implantable RVAD designed for short-term support.[104] The inflow cage is implanted in the right atrium. The flexible, ring-reinforced PTFE outflow graft is anastomosed end-to-side to the pulmonary artery. A microaxial-flow pump with a miniaturized propeller located within the inflow cannula (outer diameter 6.4 mm, 12-mL inner volume, 65-cm² blood-contacting surface, 11 g) rotates at up to 32,000 rpm to generate up to 6 L/min of blood flow (**Fig. 10**). An

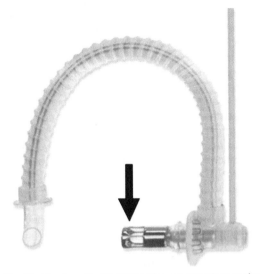

Fig. 10. The Impella RD RVAD. The arrow points to the inflow cannula that is positioned in the right atrium. The outflow graft is sewn to the pulmonary artery. (*From* Christiansen S, Perez-Bouza A, Reul, H, et al. In vivo experimental testing of a microaxial blood pump for right ventricular support. Artif Organs 2006;30:94–100; with permission.)

external purger continuously delivers in situ anticoagulation of the pump via heparinized rinsing fluid (10%–20% glucose, 2500 IU heparin at 200–600 IU heparin/h) from an external 50-mL syringe. The implantation technique is rapid, does not require cardiopulmonary bypass, additional cutaneous incisions for cannulas or a driveline, and the pump fits within the pericardium. Maximum recommended use is 10 days.[15] A pressure sensor that measures the pressure gradient across the impeller and the rotational speed are used to estimate pump flow.[104] The driveline is externalized and connected to a mobile console.

In an acute porcine model of delayed orthotopic heart transplantation–induced right ventricular failure (24-hour cold ischemic time), the Impella RD provided continuous blood flow for 5 hours.[105] Mechanical support of the left ventricle was not necessary. After weaning and explanting the device, hemodynamics remained stable. In a chronic ovine model without anticoagulation, the Impella RD successfully supported normal animals for 7 days without hemodynamic or end-organ complications.[106] Small clots were observed on the right atrial inflow cage and indicated that anticoagulation therapy is necessary with this device.

Multiple case studies and a few small case series have documented successful implementation of the Impella Recover RD as a bridge to right ventricular recovery. Although a large clinical trial has not been performed, the device has been used to support right ventricular failure after posttransplant cardiogenic shock, left ventricular rupture, repeat mitral valve replacement, LVAD implantation, and during myocardial revascularization with and without cardiopulmonary bypass.[15,104,107–111]

Impella RP

Perhaps the most exciting advance in right ventricular support is the development of the Impella Right Peripheral (Impella RP; Abiomed Incorporated, Danvers, MA, USA), a catheter-based continuous-flow device placed percutaneously via the femoral vein across the pulmonic valve. The Impella RP functions similarly to the predicate catheter-based, Abiomed Impella LP, which was designed for left heart support during high-risk PCI.[112] The inflow portion of the catheter resides within the right atrium. The outflow portion of the device resides within the main pulmonary artery.

The Impella RP has been used successfully for right-sided support after an orthotopic heart transplantation (personal communication, Anson Cheung, MD, 2011). After percutaneous placement, the Impella RP provided right ventricular support for 6 days and facilitated right ventricular recovery and explantation of the device.

Advantages of a catheter-based approach to right ventricular support include percutaneous implantation, no anastomosis, no concern for device fit, and the ability to remove the device without (re)entering the chest. If late right ventricular failure occurs, the Impella RP may be placed at the bedside without the need to transport an ill patient back to the operating room.

TAHs

Despite recent advancements in mechanical circulatory support devices, the management of biventricular failure continues to be a challenge. Although survival with LVADs continues to improve, there remains significant early morbidity and mortality caused by right ventricular failure.[22,23] In select patients, a TAH may be the best treatment option. In the past 4 decades, 14 different TAHs have been implanted globally at more than 30 centers in 1108 patients.[24] Currently, 2 TAHs are available for clinical use in the United States, the SynCardia CardioWest and the Abiomed AbioCor. However, a major limitation is the large size of these devices, which cannot be implanted in a substantial portion of the population. CardioWest implantation is limited to adult patients with a body surface area (BSA) between

1.7 and 2.5 m^2,[113] and the AbioCor does not fit in patients with a BSA less than 2.0 m^2.[114] Consequently, modifications to the CardioWest and development of the AbioCor II are underway to reduce the size of each device and expand the potential patient population.

The shift from volume displacement pumps to continuous-flow devices has progressively decreased the size and increased the durability of LVADs. The development of a continuous-flow TAH (CFTAH) is underway. As an alternative, to the TAH concurrent implantation of small, right-sided and left-sided, continuous-flow devices has evolved into a practicable therapy. The remainder of this review focuses on changes to the clinically approved CardioWest, the AbioCor II, and the Cleveland Heart CFTAH. Preliminary success and long-term feasibility of continuous-flow BiVAD therapy is examined as an emerging treatment of end-stage biventricular failure.

CardioWest

The CardioWest TAH (SynCardia Systems Incorporated, Tucson, AZ) is the world's first and only TAH approved by FDA, Health Canada, and Conformite Europeenne (CE). Available in the United States as a bridge-to-transplant therapy, the CardioWest TAH has shown better survival to transplantation than with medical management alone.[113]

The recent development of the 6.1-kg (13.5-lb) Freedom portable driver (**Fig. 11**A), which is substantially smaller than the original Big Blue driver (see **Fig. 11**B), has expanded the usefulness of the CardioWest in the United States. An IDE clinical trial is currently underway in which patients may now be discharged from the hospital. In addition, a smaller device that will fit in most adult patients is currently being developed. Trileaflet polymer, central-flow valves have replaced current tilting-disk, Medtronic-Hall valves. Also, the pneumatic membranes have been replaced by Elast-Eon, a more durable elastic polymer. The smaller CardioWest 2 will be available in 2 sizes: 70 cm^3 for patients with a BSA of 1.7 m^2 or greater and 50 cm^3 for women and patients of smaller stature with a BSA of 1.2 to 1.7 m^2. SynCardia plans to make submissions to the FDA and CE during 2011. Preclinical studies to support an IDE are underway.

AbioCor

The AbioCor TAH (Abiomed Incorporated, Danvers, MA) is approved for destination therapy in transplant-ineligible patients with severe biventricular failure. In the initial trial, 15 patients showed 30-day survival of 87% and 60-day survival of 73%.[24] The AbioCor II, a hybrid design of the AbioCor and the Penn State TAH, has been developed. The device is significantly smaller than the AbioCor and will likely have improved durability. Clinical trials have not been planned.

The AbioCor TAH is totally implantable. A major lesson learned from this experience was that TET was simple, improved patient sense-of-freedom, and did not present technical or clinical challenges. The power requirements of the AbioCor are greater than current continuous-flow LVADs, which suggests that TET technology plus a next-generation internal battery may provide prolonged periods of untethered mobility, improved quality of life, and increased acceptance by patients and referring physicians.

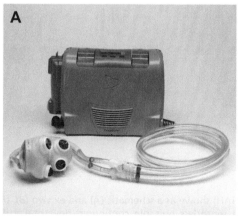
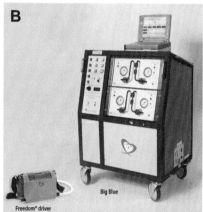

Fig. 11. The SynCardia TAH shown with the new Freedom portable driver (*A*). The Freedom portable driver is placed next to Big Blue, the old pneumatic driver (*B*). (*Courtesy of* SynCardia Systems Inc. (Tucson, AZ); with permission.)

CFTAH

The CFTAH (Cleveland Heart, Charlotte, NC) is a small (60 × 100 mm, 37 mL priming volume), valveless, sensorless, biventricular support device (**Fig. 12**A, B). The double centrifugal pump includes a single continuously rotating, brushless direct-current motor and a single rotor supported by hydrodynamic bearings. Two separate impellers are mounted on opposite ends of the rotor and create opposing forces at opposite ends of the device. A pressure regulator passively balances right-sided and left-sided pressures and flow. Within the housing, the motor's magnetic assembly is shorter than the housing laminations and allows free axial movement of the rotor from left to right. As a result, atrial pressure differences move the rotor and change the aperture at the outer diameter of the right-sided impeller to affect relative right-left output in a direction to correct right-left imbalance.[115] The control algorithm permits active speed modulation as an additional method to maintain left-right balance and induce pulsatility.

The CFTAH is designed to provide 3 to 8 L/min of flow against a systemic vascular resistance (SVR) of 700 to 2000 dyne/s/cm^{-5} and pulmonary vascular resistance (PVR) of 100 to 500 dyne/s/cm^{-5}. In a mock circulatory loop, passive self-regulation maintained balanced pump flows with atrial pressure differences of less than 10 mm Hg at physiologic and supraphysiologic PVR and SVR.[115] The CFTAH consumed 13 W at 8 L/min with 20 mm Hg and 80 mm Hg of right and left afterload, respectively.[12] The magnitude of induced pulsatility permitted active control to adjust right-left balance and pump flows and achieve a pulse pressure of 38 mm Hg. The

additional power consumption to generate a physiologic pulse pressure was 16.2%.[116]

In an acute bovine model, with rotational speeds of 2000 to 3000 rpm, the CFTAH balanced right and left flows and maintained a maximum atrial pressure difference of 10 mm Hg. By varying the amplitude of the speed waveform, the CFTAH achieved a pulse pressure of 9 mm Hg in the pulmonary artery and 18 mm Hg in the aorta.[12]

Continuous-flow BiVAD

The use of continuous-flow BiVADs as total heart replacement is gaining momentum as an attractive therapy for end-stage biventricular failure. Small, continuous-flow devices address the size and durability limitations of pulsatile systems. Importantly, left-right balance may not be an issue with this approach.

Preliminary acute animal studies have shown the feasibility of continuous-flow BiVAD with or without native cardiectomy. In an ovine model of biventriculectomy, 2 HeartMate III centrifugal assist devices satisfactorily preserved a physiologic circulation.[43] The inflow sewing rings were attached to a rim of right and left ventricular tissue. Outflow grafts were anastomosed end to end to the aorta and pulmonary artery. To balance different right and left ventricular preload and output, a large atrial-septal window was created surgically. At low RVAD speeds, the interatrial shunt was right to left. As the right-sided ventricular assist device increased speed, the interatrial shunt became bidirectional and then reversed to left to right. At no pump speed did either atrium collapse.

Subsequent experiments have shown than an interatrial shunt is unnecessary to maintain

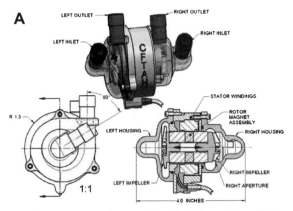
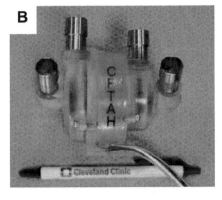

Fig. 12. The continuous-flow total artificial heart (CFTAH) shown as a schematic (*A*) and ex vivo (*B*). (*From* Fukamachi K, Horvath DJ, Massiello AL, et al. An innovative, sensorless, pulsatile, continuous-flow total artificial heart: device design and initial in vitro study. J Heart Lung Transplant 2010;29(1):13–20; with permission; and Fumoto H, Horvath DJ, Rao S, et al. In vivo acute performance of the Cleveland Clinic self-regulating, continuous-flow total artificial heart. J Heart Lung Transplant 2010;29(1):21–6; with permission.)

right-left balance during continuous-flow BiVAD support.[103,117] Unlike pulsatile flow devices, rotary pumps operate with a Starling-like response. Pump output is sensitive to both preload and afterload.[55,117] Consequently, modifications must be made to existing LVADs for use as an RVAD. Devices implanted in the left ventricle and right ventricle and set at the same speed generate different flow rates because of differences in right and left ventricular filling pressures and differences in vascular resistance. Decreasing the speed of the RVAD decreases right-sided output. However, low speeds may promote thrombosis and are not suggested.[25] A better solution may be to equalize left and right device resistance. Narrowing of the right-sided outflow graft with Prolene suture increases the resistance of the right pump to a value comparable with SVR[25] to balance the pressure/flow relationship. Of note, caution must be used when increasing the rotational speed of the RVAD. Left atrial pressure is especially sensitive to RVAD speeds, whereas right atrial pressure is less sensitive to a change in LVAD speed.[103]

Chronic large animal studies have been performed to investigate the feasibility and long-term effects of a totally pulseless circulation during total heart replacement with dual intracorporeal continuous-flow devices. In a chronic bovine model, after excision of the native heart, 2 Heart-Mate II axial-flow LVADs were implanted to replace the right and left ventricles (**Fig. 13**).[117]

During a 7-week study, nonpulsatile systemic arterial and pulmonary arterial blood flow did not adversely affect homeostasis, end-organ and vasomotor function, or the ability to exercise.[117] Right-sided and left-sided balance was achieved with right atrial pressures from 5 to 15 mm Hg. In a similar experiment, after native cardiectomy, 2 Jarvik 2000 pumps adequately maintained systemic and pulmonary circulation in a calf for 20 days.[44] Systemic and pulmonary resistances were maintained pharmacologically to preserve a mean arterial pressure of 100 mm Hg, mean pulmonary pressure of 20 mm Hg, and atrial pressures of 15 mm Hg. The left pump, set at a fixed speed of 14,000 rpm, autoregulated in response to changes in right-sided output, pulmonary and systemic pressures, activity level, and fluid status. Hemodynamics, end-organ function, and neurohormonal status remained normal throughout the study.

Initial human experiences with dual intracorporeal rotary pumps for the treatment of biventricular failure are encouraging (**Fig. 14**).[25,92,118–120] Multiple recent reports document successful implantation of dual HeartWare HVADs in patients for periods of up to 180 days without adverse events.[118] In these patients, to avoid overflowing the pulmonary circuit, the outflow graft of the right-sided pump was narrowed from 10 mm to 5 mm. In one case, a small male patient (BSA 1.6 m² and small chest size) was discharged home with an ongoing follow-up of 189 days.[119]

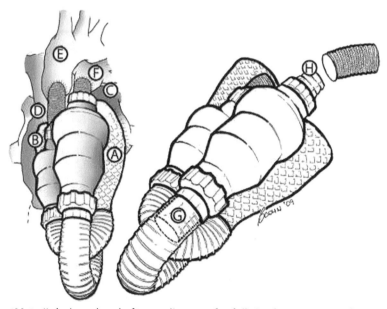

Fig. 13. Two HeartMate II devices placed after cardiectomy for full circulatory support. (*From* Frazier OH, Cohn WE, Tuzun E, et al. Continuous-flow total artificial heart supports long-term survival of a calf. Tex Heart Inst J 2009;36:568–74; with permission.)

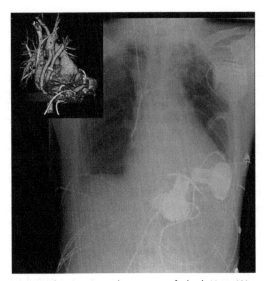

Fig. 14. The in vivo placement of dual HeartWare HVAD devices as an RVAD and an LVAD for long-term biventricular support. (*From* Loforte A, Montalto A, Della Monica PL, et al. Biventricular support with the HeartWare implantable continuous flow pump: an additional contribution. J Heart Lung Transplant 2010;29:1443–4; with permission.)

In patients with pulmonary hypertension (and an increased PVR), the RVAD outflow graft should be narrowed to a lesser degree to ensure comparable PVR and SVR.[25] It remains to be determined whether dual continuous-flow pumps may increase the susceptibility, compared with a single continuous-flow LVAD, to acquired von Willebrand disease and bleeding events.[121] One controller and 1 battery source for both devices remains to be developed.

SUMMARY

Recent international experience with continuous-flow devices has progressively improved clinical outcomes and the quality of life of patients who require mechanical circulatory support to survive. New databanks for implantable cardiac devices such as INTERMACS will increase this trend. As devices are miniaturized for earlier support with less-invasive operative approaches, the incidence and prevalence of long-term mechanical circulatory support is likely to increase globally.

Novel LVADs, RVADs, BiVADs, and TAHs should reduce the problems of present systems. The implantation, operation, and management profiles of next-generation devices will be different from each other and different from predicate devices. Less-invasive surgical approaches and strategies of long-term partial unloading of the heart must be further investigated and refined.

Invasive full-support devices may still be reserved as a final treatment option for patients with life-threatening, end-stage heart failure as a bridge to heart transplantation or as a destination therapy. In contrast, less-invasive partial-support devices may prove successful for the management of less-severe heart failure and relieve heart transplantation waiting lists. Partial-support devices may interrupt the progressive hemodynamic deterioration of heart failure, improve symptoms and quality of life, promote reverse myocardial remodeling, and allow for device explantation in select patients. Smaller TAHs and dual intracorporeal rotary pumps may expand the treatment options for patients with end-stage biventricular failure.

Proper patient selection is critical to achieving success with any device and should be tailored to patient needs. Ultimately, careful examination of experiences with future generations of implantable devices will determine the relative usefulness for each device.

REFERENCES

1. Mielniczuk L, Mussivand T, Davies R, et al. Patient selection for left ventricular assist devices. Artif Organs 2004;28:152–7.
2. Eurotransplant. Eurotransplant Annual Report. Available at: www.eurotransplant.nl. Accessed January 2011.
3. Stehlik J, Edwards LB, Kucheryavaya AY, et al. The Registry of the International Society for Heart and Lung Transplantation: twenty-seventh official adult heart transplant report–2010. J Heart Lung Transplant 2010;29:1089–103.
4. Farrar DJ, Bourque K, Dague CP, et al. Design features, developmental status, and experimental results with the HeartMate III centrifugal left ventricular assist system with a magnetically levitated rotor. ASAIO J 2007;53:310–5.
5. Slaughter MS, Sobieski MA 2nd, Tamez D, et al. HeartWare miniature axial-flow ventricular assist device: design and initial feasibility test. Tex Heart Inst J 2009;36:12–6.
6. Hoshi H, Shinshi T, Takatani S. Third-generation blood pumps with mechanical noncontact magnetic bearings. Artif Organs 2006;30:324–38.
7. Meyns BP, Simon A, Klotz S, et al. Clinical benefits of partial circulatory support in New York Heart Association class IIIB and early class IV patients. Eur J Cardiothorac Surg 2011;39(5):693–8.
8. Bartoli CR, Wilson GC, Giridharan GA, et al. A novel subcutaneous counterpulsation device: acute hemodynamic efficacy during pharmacologically induced hypertension, hypotension, and heart failure. Artif Organs 2010;34:537–45.

9. Sales VL, McCarthy PM. Understanding the C-pulse device and its potential to treat heart failure. Curr Heart Fail Rep 2010;7:27–34.

10. Smith EJ, Reitan O, Keeble T, et al. A first-in-man study of the Reitan catheter pump for circulatory support in patients undergoing high-risk percutaneous coronary intervention. Catheter Cardiovasc Interv 2009;73:859–65.

11. Baldwin JT, Borovetz HS, Duncan BW, et al. The National Heart, Lung, and Blood Institute Pediatric Circulatory Support Program. Circulation 2006;113:147–55.

12. Fumoto H, Horvath DJ, Rao S, et al. In vivo acute performance of the Cleveland Clinic self-regulating, continuous-flow total artificial heart. J Heart Lung Transplant 2010;29:21–6.

13. Fukamachi K, Saeed D, Massiello AL, et al. Development of DexAide right ventricular assist device: update II. ASAIO J 2008;54:589–93.

14. Gazzoli F, Alloni A, Pagani F, et al. Arrow CorAide left ventricular assist system: initial experience of the cardio-thoracic surgery center in Pavia. Ann Thorac Surg 2007;83:279–82.

15. Sugiki H, Nakashima K, Vermes E, et al. Temporary right ventricular support with Impella Recover RD axial flow pump. Asian Cardiovasc Thorac Ann 2009;17:395–400.

16. Krishnamani R, DeNofrio D, Konstam MA. Emerging ventricular assist devices for long-term cardiac support. Nat Rev Cardiol 2010;7:71–6.

17. Jeevanandam V, Jayakar D, Anderson AS, et al. Circulatory assistance with a permanent implantable IABP: initial human experience. Circulation 2002;106:I183–8.

18. Yamazaki K, et al. Next generation LVAD "EVA-HEART": current status of Japanese clinical trial. J Card Fail 2006;12(Suppl).

19. Meyns B, Klotz S, Simon A, et al. Proof of concept: hemodynamic response to long-term partial ventricular support with the Synergy Pocket Micro-Pump. J Am Coll Cardiol 2009;54:79–86.

20. Hayward CS, Peters WS, Merry AF, et al. Chronic extra-aortic balloon counterpulsation: first-in-human pilot study in end-stage heart failure. J Heart Lung Transplant 2010;29:1427–32.

21. Kaul TK, Fields BL. Postoperative acute refractory right ventricular failure: incidence, pathogenesis, management and prognosis. Cardiovasc Surg 2000;8:1–9.

22. Potapov EV, Loforte A, Weng Y, et al. Experience with over 1000 implanted ventricular assist devices. J Card Surg 2008;23:185–94.

23. Kavarana MN, Pessin-Minsley MS, Urtecho J, et al. Right ventricular dysfunction and organ failure in left ventricular assist device recipients: a continuing problem. Ann Thorac Surg 2002;73:745–50.

24. Bartoli CR, Anderson M, Dowling RD. The total artificial heart: bridge-to-transplant and destination-therapy for end-stage biventricular heart failure. Philadelphia: Lippincott Williams & Wilkins; 2010.

25. Hetzer R, Krabatsch T, Stepanenko A, et al. Long-term biventricular support with the heartware implantable continuous flow pump. J Heart Lung Transplant 2010;29:822–4.

26. Goldstein DJ, Oz MC, Rose EA. Implantable left ventricular assist devices. N Engl J Med 1998;339:1522–33.

27. Rose EA, Gelijns AC, Moskowitz AJ, et al. Long-term mechanical left ventricular assistance for end-stage heart failure. N Engl J Med 2001;345:1435–43.

28. Slaughter MS, Rogers JG, Milano CA, et al. Advanced heart failure treated with continuous-flow left ventricular assist device. N Engl J Med 2009;361(23):2241–51.

29. Birks EJ, Yacoub MH, Banner NR, et al. The role of bridge to transplantation: should LVAD patients be transplanted? Curr Opin Cardiol 2004;19:148–53.

30. Birks EJ, Tansley PD, Hardy J, et al. Left ventricular assist device and drug therapy for the reversal of heart failure. N Engl J Med 2006;355:1873–84.

31. Frazier OH, Myers TJ. Left ventricular assist system as a bridge to myocardial recovery. Ann Thorac Surg 1999;68:734–41.

32. Reitz BA. Mechanical devices and US Food and Drug Administration (FDA) approval. Semin Thorac Cardiovasc Surg Pediatr Card Surg Annu 2006;123–7.

33. Bartoli CR, Giridharan GA, Litwak KN, et al. Hemodynamic responses to continuous versus pulsatile mechanical unloading of the failing left ventricle. ASAIO J 2010;56(5):410–6.

34. Thoratec. Thoratec announces filing of PMA seeking destination therapy approval for HeartMate II [press release]. 2009.

35. FDA. Thoratec HeartMate II LVAS - P060040/S005 [press release]. 2010.

36. Kirklin JK, Naftel DC, Kormos RL, et al. Third INTERMACS Annual Report: the evolution of destination therapy in the United States. J Heart Lung Transplant 2011;30:115–23.

37. Bourque K, Dague C, Farrar D, et al. In vivo assessment of a rotary left ventricular assist device-induced artificial pulse in the proximal and distal aorta. Artif Organs 2006;30:638–42.

38. Khalil HA, Kerr DT, Schusterman MA 2nd, et al. Induced pulsation of a continuous-flow total artificial heart in a mock circulatory system. J Heart Lung Transplant 2010;29:568–73.

39. Menconi MJ, Pockwinse S, Owen TA, et al. Properties of blood-contacting surfaces of clinically implanted cardiac assist devices: gene expression,

matrix composition, and ultrastructural characterization of cellular linings. J Cell Biochem 1995;57: 557–73.

40. Slaughter MS, Myers TJ. Transcutaneous energy transmission for mechanical circulatory support systems: history, current status, and future prospects. J Card Surg 2010;25:484–9.

41. Bourque K, Gernes DB, Loree HM 2nd, et al. HeartMate III: pump design for a centrifugal LVAD with a magnetically levitated rotor. ASAIO J 2001;47: 401–5.

42. Slaughter MS, Bartoli CR, Sobieski MA, et al. Intraoperative evaluation of the HeartMate II Flow Estimator. J Heart Lung Transplant 2009;28: 39–43.

43. Frazier OH, Tuzun E, Cohn W, et al. Total heart replacement with dual centrifugal ventricular assist devices. ASAIO J 2005;51:224–9.

44. Frazier OH, Tuzun E, Cohn WE, et al. Total heart replacement using dual intracorporeal continuous-flow pumps in a chronic bovine model: a feasibility study. ASAIO J 2006;52:145–9.

45. Takaseya T, Fumoto H, Shiose A, et al. In vivo biocompatibility evaluation of a new resilient, hard-carbon, thin-film coating for ventricular assist devices. Artif Organs 2010;34:1158–63.

46. Gerhart RL, Horvath DJ, Ochiai Y, et al. The effects of impact on the CorAide ventricular assist device. ASAIO J 2002;48:449–52.

47. Doi K, Golding LA, Massiello AL, et al. Preclinical readiness testing of the Arrow International CorAide left ventricular assist system. Ann Thorac Surg 2004;77:2103–10.

48. Fukamachi K. New technologies for mechanical circulatory support: current status and future prospects of CorAide and MagScrew technologies. J Artif Organs 2004;7:45–57.

49. Fukamachi K, Ochiai Y, Doi K, et al. Chronic evaluation of the Cleveland Clinic CorAide left ventricular assist system in calves. Artif Organs 2002; 26:529–33.

50. Ochiai Y, Golding LA, Massiello AL, et al. Cleveland clinic CorAide blood pump circulatory support without anticoagulation. ASAIO J 2002;48:249–52.

51. Yamazaki K, Kihara S, Akimoto T, et al. EVAHEART: an implantable centrifugal blood pump for long-term circulatory support. Jpn J Thorac Cardiovasc Surg 2002;50:461–5.

52. Kihara S, Yamazaki K, Litwak KN, et al. In vivo evaluation of a MPC polymer coated continuous flow left ventricular assist system. Artif Organs 2003; 27:188–92.

53. Snyder TA, Tsukui H, Kihara S, et al. Preclinical biocompatibility assessment of the EVAHEART ventricular assist device: coating comparison and platelet activation. J Biomed Mater Res A 2007; 81:85–92.

54. Yamazaki K, Mori T, Tomioka J, et al. The cool seal system: a practical solution to the shaft seal problem and heat related complications with implantable rotary blood pumps. ASAIO J 1997; 43:M567–71.

55. Akimoto T, Yamazaki K, Litwak P, et al. Rotary blood pump flow spontaneously increases during exercise under constant pump speed: results of a chronic study. Artif Organs 1999;23:797–801.

56. Yamazaki K, Saito S, Kihara S, et al. Completely pulsatile high flow circulatory support with a constant-speed centrifugal blood pump: mechanisms and early clinical observations. Gen Thorac Cardiovasc Surg 2007;55:158–62.

57. Casula R, Athanasiou T, Foale R. Recent advances in minimal-access cardiac surgery using robotic-enhanced surgical systems. Expert Rev Cardiovasc Ther 2004;2:589–600.

58. Frazier OH. Implantation of the Jarvik 2000 left ventricular assist device without the use of cardiopulmonary bypass. Ann Thorac Surg 2003; 75:1028–30.

59. Hunt SA. Mechanical circulatory support: new data, old problems. Circulation 2007;116:461–2.

60. HeartWare. MVAD and HVAD Update - HeartWare International, Inc. Available at: http://202.66.146.82/listco/au/heartware/cpresent/cpr081120.pdf. Accessed January 2011.

61. Baldwin JT, Mann DL. NHLBI's program for VAD therapy for moderately advanced heart failure: the REVIVE-IT pilot trial. J Card Fail 2010;16:855–8.

62. Morley D, Litwak K, Ferber P, et al. Hemodynamic effects of partial ventricular support in chronic heart failure: results of simulation validated with in vivo data. J Thorac Cardiovasc Surg 2007;133:21–8.

63. Burkhoff D, Klotz S, Mancini DM. LVAD-induced reverse remodeling: basic and clinical implications for myocardial recovery. J Card Fail 2006;12:227–39.

64. Entwistle JW 3rd. Short- and long-term mechanical ventricular assistance towards myocardial recovery. Surg Clin N Am 2004;84:201–21.

65. Birks EJ, George RS. Molecular changes occurring during reverse remodelling following left ventricular assist device support. J Cardiovasc Transl Res 2010;3:635–42.

66. Kinoshita M, Takano H, Taenaka Y, et al. Cardiac disuse atrophy during LVAD pumping. ASAIO Trans 1988;34:208–12.

67. Kinoshita M, Takano H, Takaichi S, et al. Influence of prolonged ventricular assistance on myocardial histopathology in intact heart. Ann Thorac Surg 1996;61:640–5.

68. Klotz S, Foronjy RF, Dickstein ML, et al. Mechanical unloading during left ventricular assist device support increases left ventricular collagen cross-linking and myocardial stiffness. Circulation 2005; 112:364–74.

69. Rose AG, Park SJ. Pathology in patients with ventricular assist devices: a study of 21 autopsies, 24 ventricular apical core biopsies and 24 explanted hearts. Cardiovasc Pathol 2005;14:19–23.

70. Ziv O, Dizon J, Thosani A, et al. Effects of left ventricular assist device therapy on ventricular arrhythmias. J Am Coll Cardiol 2005;45:1428–34.

71. Vollkron M, Voitl P, Ta J, et al. Suction events during left ventricular support and ventricular arrhythmias. J Heart Lung Transplant 2007;26:819–25.

72. Vandenberghe S, Nishida T, Segers P, et al. The impact of pump speed and inlet cannulation site on left ventricular unloading with a rotary blood pump. Artif Organs 2004;28:660–7.

73. Klotz S, Meyns B, Simon A, et al. Partial mechanical long-term support with the CircuLite Synergy Pump as bridge-to-transplant in congestive heart failure. Thorac Cardiovasc Surg 2010;58(Suppl 2): S173–8.

74. Reitan O, Sternby J, Ohlin H. Hydrodynamic properties of a new percutaneous intra-aortic axial flow pump. ASAIO J 2000;46:323–9.

75. Reitan O, Ohlin H, Peterzén B, et al. Initial tests with a new cardiac assist device. ASAIO J 1999;45: 317–21.

76. Dekker A, Reesink K, van der Veen E, et al. Efficacy of a new intraaortic propeller pump vs the intra-aortic balloon pump: an animal study. Chest 2003;123:2089–95.

77. Reitan O, Steen S, Ohlin H. Hemodynamic effects of a new percutaneous circulatory support device in a left ventricular failure model. ASAIO J 2003; 49:731–6.

78. Manord JD, Garrard CL, Mehra MR, et al. Implications for the vascular surgeon with prolonged (3 to 89 days) intraaortic balloon pump counterpulsation. J Vasc Surg 1997;26:511–5 [discussion: 515–6].

79. Freed PS, Wasfie T, Zado B, et al. Intraaortic balloon pumping for prolonged circulatory support. Am J Cardiol 1988;61:554–7.

80. Sherwood JT, Schomisch SJ, Thompson DR, et al. Aortomyoplasty: hemodynamics and comparison to the intraaortic balloon pump. J Surg Res 2003; 110:315–21.

81. Patel BG, Shah SH, Astra LI, et al. Skeletal muscle ventricle aortic counterpulsation: function during chronic heart failure. Ann Thorac Surg 2002;73: 588–93.

82. Terrovitis JV, Charitos CE, Tsolakis EJ, et al. Superior performance of a paraaortic counterpulsation device compared to the intraaortic balloon pump. World J Surg 2003;27:1311–6.

83. Davies AN, Peters WS, Su T, et al. Extra-ascending aortic versus intra-descending aortic balloon counterpulsation-effect on coronary artery blood flow. Heart Lung Circ 2005;14:178–86.

84. Legget ME, Peters WS, Milsom FP, et al. Extra-aortic balloon counterpulsation: an intraoperative feasibility study. Circulation 2005;112:I26–31.

85. Mitnovetski S, Almeida AA, Barr A, et al. Extra-aortic implantable counterpulsation pump in chronic heart failure. Ann Thorac Surg 2008;85:2122–5.

86. Giridharan GA, Pantalos GM, Litwak KN, et al. Predicted hemodynamic benefits of counterpulsation therapy using a superficial surgical approach. ASAIO J 2006;52:39–46.

87. Koenig SC, Pantalos GM, Litwak KN, et al. Hemodynamic and left ventricular pressure-volume responses to counterpulsation in mock circulation and acute large animal models. Conf Proc IEEE Eng Med Biol Soc 2004;5:3761–4.

88. Trost JC, Hillis LD. Intra-aortic balloon counterpulsation. Am J Cardiol 2006;97:1391–8.

89. Koenig SC, Spence PA, Pantalos GM, et al. Development and early testing of a simple subcutaneous counterpulsation device. ASAIO J 2006;52:362–7.

90. Koenig SC, Litwak KN, Giridharan GA, et al. Acute hemodynamic efficacy of a 32-ml subcutaneous counterpulsation device in a calf model of diminished cardiac function. ASAIO J 2008;54:578–84.

91. Moskowitz A, Williams D, Tierney A, et al. Economic Considerations of Left Ventricular Assist Device (LVAD) Implantation. In: Oz M, Goldstein D, editors. Cardiac Assist Devices. Armonk (NY): Futura Publishing Company, Inc; 1999.

92. Frazier OH, Myers TJ, Gregoric I. Biventricular assistance with the Jarvik FlowMaker: a case report. J Thorac Cardiovasc Surg 2004;128:625–6.

93. Reichenbach SH, Farrar DJ, Hill JD. A versatile intracorporeal ventricular assist device based on the Thoratec VAD system. Ann Thorac Surg 2001;71: S171–5 [discussion: S183–4].

94. Moazami N, Pasque MK, Moon MR, et al. Mechanical support for isolated right ventricular failure in patients after cardiotomy. J Heart Lung Transplant 2004;23:1371–5.

95. Fukamachi K, Ootaki Y, Horvath DJ, et al. Progress in the development of the DexAide right ventricular assist device. ASAIO J 2006;52:630–3.

96. Saeed D, Horvath DJ, Massiello AL, et al. Use of zirconia ceramic in the DexAide right ventricular assist device journal bearing. Artif Organs 2010; 34:146–9.

97. Fukamachi K, Horvath DJ, Massiello AL, et al. Development of a small implantable right ventricular assist device. ASAIO J 2005;51:730–5.

98. Ootaki Y, Saeed D, Ootaki C, et al. Development of the DexAide right ventricular assist device inflow cannula. ASAIO J 2008;54:31–6.

99. Saeed D, Shalli S, Fumoto H, et al. In vivo evaluation of zirconia ceramic in the DexAide right ventricular assist device journal bearing. Artif Organs 2010;34:512–6.

100. Saeed D, Massiello AL, Shalli S, et al. Introduction of fixed-flow mode in the DexAide right ventricular assist device. J Heart Lung Transplant 2010;29: 32–6.

101. Ootaki Y, Ootaki C, Kamohara K, et al. Cadaver fitting study of the DexAide right ventricular assist device. Artif Organs 2007;31:646–8.

102. Ootaki Y, Ootaki C, Massiello A, et al. Human clinical fitting study of the DexAide right ventricular assist device. Artif Organs 2009;33:558–61.

103. Saeed D, Ootaki Y, Ootaki C, et al. Acute in vivo evaluation of an implantable continuous flow biventricular assist system. ASAIO J 2008;54:20–4.

104. Christiansen S, Dohmen G, Autschbach R. Treatment of right heart failure with a new microaxial blood pump. Asian Cardiovasc Thorac Ann 2006; 14:418–21.

105. Martin J, Benk C, Yerebakan C, et al. The new "Impella" intracardiac microaxial pump for treatment of right heart failure after orthotopic heart transplantation. Transplant Proc 2001;33:3549–50.

106. Christiansen S, Perez-Bouza A, Reul H, et al. In vivo experimental testing of a microaxial blood pump for right ventricular support. Artif Organs 2006;30:94–100.

107. Schmidt T, Siefker J, Spiliopoulos S, et al. New experience with the paracardial right ventricular axial flow micropump Impella Elect 600. Eur J Cardiothorac Surg 2003;24:307–8.

108. Jurmann MJ, Siniawski H, Erb M, et al. Initial experience with miniature axial flow ventricular assist devices for postcardiotomy heart failure. Ann Thorac Surg 2004;77:1642–7.

109. Christiansen S, Brose S, Demircan L, et al. A new right ventricular assist device for right ventricular support. Eur J Cardiothorac Surg 2003;24:834–6.

110. Boening A, Friedrich C, Caliebe D, et al. Efficacy of intracardiac right ventricular microaxial pump support during beating heart surgery. Interact Cardiovasc Thorac Surg 2004;3:495–8.

111. Lamarche Y, Cheung A, Ignaszewski A, et al. Comparative outcomes in cardiogenic shock patients managed with Impella microaxial pump or extracorporeal life support. J Thorac Cardiovasc Surg 2011;142(1):60–5.

112. Engstrom AE, Piek JJ, Henriques JP. Percutaneous left ventricular assist devices for high-risk percutaneous coronary intervention. Expert Rev Cardiovasc Ther 2010;8:1247–55.

113. Copeland JG, Smith RG, Arabia FA, et al. Cardiac replacement with a total artificial heart as a bridge to transplantation. N Engl J Med 2004;351:859–67.

114. Samuels LE, Dowling R. Total artificial heart: destination therapy. Cardiol Clin 2003;21:115–8.

115. Fukamachi K, Horvath DJ, Massiello AL, et al. An innovative, sensorless, pulsatile, continuous-flow total artificial heart: device design and initial in vitro study. J Heart Lung Transplant 2010;29: 13–20.

116. Shiose A, Nowak K, Horvath DJ, et al. Speed modulation of the continuous-flow total artificial heart to simulate a physiologic arterial pressure waveform. ASAIO J 2010;56:403–9.

117. Frazier OH, Cohn WE, Tuzun E, et al. Continuous-flow total artificial heart supports long-term survival of a calf. Tex Heart Inst J 2009;36:568–74.

118. Strueber M, Meyer AL, Malehsa D, et al. Successful use of the HeartWare HVAD rotary blood pump for biventricular support. J Thorac Cardiovasc Surg 2010;140:936–7.

119. Loforte A, Lilla Della Monica P, Montalto A, et al. HeartWare third-generation implantable continuous flow pump as biventricular support: midterm follow-up. Interact Cardiovasc Thorac Surg 2011;12(3):458–60.

120. Loforte A, Montalto A, Della Monica PL, et al. Biventricular support with the HeartWare implantable continuous flow pump: an additional contribution. J Heart Lung Transplant 2010;29:1443–4.

121. Geisen U, Heilmann C, Beyersdorf F, et al. Non-surgical bleeding in patients with ventricular assist devices could be explained by acquired von Willebrand disease. Eur J Cardiothorac Surg 2008;33:679–84.

Editorial Comments on "The Future of Adult Cardiac Assist Devices: Novel Systems and Mechanical Circulatory Support Strategies"

John A. Elefteriades, MD

KEY CONCEPTS

Drs Carlo R. Bartoli and Robert D. Dowling, authors of "The Future of Adult Cardiac Assist Devices: Novel Systems and Mechanical Circulatory Support Strategies," comprehensively describe imaginative novel approaches to mechanical support. Imagination and creativity are in clear evidence.

STRENGTHS

Tremendous promise is palpable in the authors' descriptions of these devices in preparation and/ or clinical testing phases.

WEAKNESSES

There is promise but no ideal device realized yet. Mechanical failure, thrombosis, hemorrhage, and problems in physiologic responsiveness and energy delivery continue to plague this exciting field.

Section of Cardiac Surgery, Yale University School of Medicine, Boardman 2, 333 Cedar Street, New Haven, CT 06510, USA
E-mail address: john.elefteriades@yale.edu

Cardiol Clin 29 (2011) 583
doi:10.1016/j.ccl.2011.07.003
0733-8651/11/$ – see front matter © 2011 Published by Elsevier Inc

Transplant or VAD?

Robert Jarvik, MD

KEYWORDS

- Vascular assist device • Heart transplant • Heart disease
- Mechanical circulatory support device

COMPARING VAD AND TRANSPLANT

The assumption was once that a heart transplant was a better choice than a mechanical circulatory support device. It is time to reconsider.

Some facts to consider are:

1. More than 20,000 patients have been treated with VADs, with the current implant rate more than double the rate of heart transplants.
2. Most VAD implants have been used as a bridge to transplant, with posttransplant survival at least equal to, if not slightly better than, that for patients transplanted without VADs.[1]
3. The longest survival for a patient with a VAD implant is 7.5 years.[2]
4. Heart transplant has a 2-year survival rate of 80% and a 5-year survival rate of 60%.[3]
5. Several leading VADs are showing a survival trend essentially the same as transplant, but there has not yet been time to evaluate survival in the 5- to 10-year time frame.[4]
6. Two-year data are available for patients undergoing implantation as destination therapy (DT) in the United States. Under the HeartMate II DT study, the 2-year survival was 58%, but the protocol required implant in only patients with advanced heart failure, and clinical practice limited use to the sickest patients early in the study.[2] As more data became available, cardiologists began to become comfortable with earlier referrals. A 1-year survival rate of 85% was seen in 169 patients followed in a postapproval bridge-to-transplant study, without any modifications to the blood pump. The reasons for this improvement likely relate to selection of less-sick candidates once the clinical community moved beyond the strict restrictions of the protocol and began to recognize the importance of earlier intervention. Additionally, the postmarket experience benefited from improved patient management as many teams increased their VAD proficiency.
7. VADs preserve the natural heart, which can recover in some cases, especially with viral cardiomyopathy and postpartum cardiomyopathy (see the article by Yacoub elsewhere in this issue). If accidental damage occurs to the external equipment, such as a cable connector crushed in a car door, the patient continues to receive flow from the natural heart and has time to replace the cable. However, the amount of time depends on the amount of backflow in the specific model VAD and the condition of the individual patient's natural heart. With the Jarvik 2000 (Jarvik Heart, Inc., New York, NY, USA), patients must pass a pump-off test before hospital discharge. In this test, the pump is turned off for 3 minutes and the patient must then change all of their external equipment (controller, cables, and batteries) to their backup equipment without assistance. The Jarvik 2000 has a mean backflow of 0.5 to 0.75 L/min when off, and almost all patients tolerate this for at least 3 minutes. The HeartMate II (Thoratec Corporation, Pleasanton, CA, USA) and HeartWare (Framingham, MA, USA) pumps both have approximately 2 L/min backflow when off and patients may become disorientated or lose consciousness within 1 or 2 minutes, and require assistance to change to the backup.
8. The major serious adverse events associated with VADs after the perioperative period are infection, bleeding, thromboembolism, and stroke. The incidence of these is decreasing with the more recent device improvements.
9. Patient quality of life has been excellent for most patients with long-term rotary VADs, with rehabilitation from New York Heart

Jarvik Heart, Inc., 333 West 52nd Street, New York, NY 10019-6238, USA
E-mail address: rgreene@jarvikheart.com

Cardiol Clin 29 (2011) 585–595
doi:10.1016/j.ccl.2011.08.001
0733-8651/11/$ – see front matter © 2011 Elsevier Inc. All rights reserved.

cardiology.theclinics.com

Association (NYHA) class IV to class I or II. Patients have freely engaged in all sorts of vigorous activities, including tennis, basketball, skiing, running, hiking, and politics.

10. Mechanical reliability of the Jarvik 2000, HeartMate II, and HeartWare pumps has been excellent, with practically no failures of the implanted components of the devices. Excellent data support their high reliability for more than a decade. Cable failures have been a problem for the HeartMate II, but the risk of failure decreased after a recall of some pumps with the early cable design. The implanted portion of the Jarvik 2000 cable has never failed, and the model using the postauricular cable exit site has a connector directly at the skin level, so that any external damage cannot affect the implant. Thus, external cable damage can immediately be corrected by replacing the external cable with a backup.

11. A total of 50,000 heart transplants have been performed in the United States. Approximately 50% of these patients survive 10 years, and approximately 16% have survived more than 20 years.

12. Approximately 50% of patients who have undergone heart transplant have one or more rejection episodes in the first postoperative year. Chronic rejection can begin years after surgery.

13. Patients who have undergone heart transplant require antirejection medications and frequent follow-up visits, including numerous heart biopsies.

14. The impact of medications on patients who have undergone heart transplant is substantial. Cyclosporin A, tacrolimus, prednisone, and sirolimus are among the commonly used drugs that have many side effects, including hypertension, diabetes, renal toxicity, hepatic toxicity, graft atherosclerosis, leukemia and other malignancies, seizures, stomach ulcers, osteoporosis, cataracts, weight gain, changed appearance of the face, increased hair growth, tremors, headache, nausea, and increased risk of common infections, such as flu, pneumonia, and fungal infections.

15. Patients with VADs require anticoagulation but no immunosuppression or antirejection drugs.

16. The cost of follow-up care for VADs is much lower than for transplant because the transplant medications and biopsy procedures are very expensive. After the first year, costs for Jarvik 2000 replacement batteries, cables, and other parts is approximately $5000 per year compared with more than $50,000 per year for transplant medications and biopsies.

17. Increasingly more patients are aware of VADs as an option, especially when they are not transplant candidates. Some bridge-to-transplant patients are deciding to stay with their VADs long term, rather than being listed for transplant.

THE TRANSITION FROM VAD THERAPY AS BRIDGE TO LONG-TERM APPLICATION

A clear distinction used to exist between bridge-to-transplant and destination therapy. But the intention to treat is becoming increasingly less differentiated, and increasingly more categories are being recognized, including bridge to recovery, bridge to transplant, destination therapy (for patients with specific contraindications to transplant), and rescue therapy.

The Interagency Registry for Mechanically Assisted Circulatory Support (INTERMACS) data through June 2010 has shown that 48% (1158/2389) of patients who received VADs as a bridge to transplant were not listed for transplant at the time of VAD implant.[5] These patients were categorized as "likely to be eligible," "moderately likely to be eligible," or "unlikely to be eligible."

Other suggested categories include lifetime use (elective use for patients who qualify for transplant but do not want transplant) and maintenance therapy (patients are supported for more than 2 years before they may receive a donor heart).

Intention to treat is an arbitrary method of categorizing patients that has more to do with regulatory and insurance issues than with physiologic and pathologic conditions of the potential patient population. In the June 10, 2010 INTERMACS registry,[5] 59 patients were treated as bridge-to-recovery, of whom 12 recovered (sufficiently to have their pump removed). But 54 other patients were categorized as bridge-to-transplant who recovered among the much larger group of all patients treated with the intention to transplant. This example illustrates that although a small group of patients with a higher-than-usual likelihood for recovery may be recognized in advance of VAD implant, recovery remains unpredictable in most patients with ischemic and idiopathic cardiomyopathy. A functionally based decision, in which VAD support is used based on hemodynamic need and freedom from contraindications, is expected to eventually replace the intention to treat categories.

DONOR ALLOCATION

The availability of donor hearts remains a severe limitation, and changes in the way organs are allocated are expected. For example, giving preference to younger patients who would receive more years of benefit from the donor hearts, and using long-term VADs in older patients with less of their natural life expectancy remaining would seem reasonable. Whatever criteria are used, societal and cost issues are expected to drive the allocation process toward the maximum benefit at the lowest cost. Based on the improved quality of life and longer survival of patients with VADs, a new method of allocating donor hearts for bridge patients could be adopted for VADs that have a 2-year survival rate as good as transplant. These patients should keep their VADs for 2 years before being listed for transplant, except in emergencies. Patients who receive transplants would then have the 2 years with their VAD as additional survival benefit together with the years they are supported by the donor heart. This way of obtaining the summed benefit of VAD and transplant, which could be called *maintenance therapy*, would logically be extended to 3, 5, and more years, as VADs prove they achieve survival equal or better than transplant.

VAD VERSUS NO TRANSPLANT

The real choice that most patients will face is the choice of a VAD or nothing, because many more patients are in need of transplant than there are donors. Currently, only the HeartMate II is approved for destination therapy, but many patients have the option to participate in clinical trials. Several VADs are undergoing clinical trials for either bridge or destination therapy, including the Jarvik 2000, HeartWare, and Levacor (World Heart Corp., Salt Lake City, UT, USA). More than one of these is usually available at cardiac surgery centers, so the individual merits of each system and the overall results of long-term VAD support must be understood.

CHARACTERISTICS OF VADS DEVELOPED FOR LONG-TERM USE

The use of positive displacement blood pumps, such as the Thoratec pneumatic pump, the HeartMate I pusher plate pump, or the short-term AB 5000 pneumatic diaphragm pump, although still clinically available, has been eclipsed by the permanent electrically powered rotary pumps.

Many characteristics differentiate among the rotary pump systems, including surgical positioning (abdominal, intrathoracic, or intraventricular); blood pump type (axial or centrifugal); bearings (mechanical/blood immersed, partial magnetic and hydrodynamic, or fully magnetic); outflow graft position (ascending aorta, or descending aorta); control approach (maximize VAD flow to decompress the natural heart, or minimize VAD flow to exercise the natural heart); controller features (flow calculation, data logging, alarms, and independent adjustment to accommodate exercise level without requiring attachment to a console); power cable type, infection susceptibility, failure susceptibility, and position (abdominal or postauricular); biomaterials, tissue integration, and flow patterns to prevent blood damage and thrombosis; backflow and thrombus risk if accidentally stopped because of external equipment damage or malfunction; fit and applicability to biventricular support; durability and reliability; quality of life, including safety, freedom from serious adverse events or rehospitalizations, ease of use, body image, interference of abdominal cables with clothing and daily activities, ability to bathe and shower, battery weight and time between recharge, and minimal need for close medical supervision and accompaniment by a trained technician/caregiver.

PATIENT CONSIDERATIONS AND FOLLOW-UP HOME CARE

Although the device manufacturers, medical staff, and clinical support team are very aware of the engineering details of each system, patients are most concerned with the degree of recovery they get, their exercise tolerance, the management of their medications, the size and weight of the external components, the battery life, and the issues requiring ongoing attention, such as personal hygiene, bathing, changing the dressings, keeping backup equipment available at all times. These factors are relatively easy to manage in most patients once they have recovered sufficiently to return home. Although taking care of themselves with mechanical blood pumps requires considerably more attention than heart transplant self-care, in most cases patients with VADs accommodate so well that they can return to many of the activities they did before developing heart failure.

SYSTEM CHARACTERISTICS OF FOUR CLINICALLY APPLIED ROTARY VADS

Table 1 compares some of the system characteristics of the Jarvik 2000, HeartWare, HeartMate II, and Levacor. Because no prospective randomized studies have been performed, it is not possible to statistically compare results, but each system has important accomplishments, including:

- The longest patient survival (7.5 years) with the Jarvik 2000

Table 1
Characteristics of four portable electrically powered VADs

	Intrathoracic vs Abdominal	Size/Weight	Safety	Quality of Life	Controller	Controller Technology	Applicable to Right Heart	Applicable to Biventricular support
Jarvik 2000	Intraventricular axial flow pump Cone bearings	Small, lightweight 30 cm³/ 90g	"Brief Pump Stop" safe	Postauricular or small abdominal cable. "No bandage" shower OK.	Mobile five-speed adjustment by patient	Analog No software	Fits well Implants ongoing	Yes
HeartWare	Thoracic centrifugal pump Hydrodynamic and magnetic bearings	Small, medium weight 50 cm³/ 142g	"Brief Pump Stop" unsafe	Small abdominal cable. Bandage required. No showering.	Adjustment requires console	Digital Requires software	Fits but requires flow constrictor	Yes, but requires flow constrictor
HeartMate II	Abdominal Axial flow pump Ball/cup bearings	Medium size and weight 114 cm³/ 340g	"Brief Pump Stop" unsafe	Stiffer abdominal cable with significant failure rate. Bandage required. No showering.	Adjustment requires console	Digital Requires software	Not used for right heart	No
Levacor	Abdominal Magnetically suspended centrifugal	Large & heavy 155 cm³/ 400g	"Brief Pump Stop" unsafe	Stiffer abdominal cable with unknown failure rate. Bandage required. No showering.	Mobile three-speed adjustment by patient	Digital Requires software	Not used for right heart	No

Desirable – green
Acceptable – blue
Less desirable - yellow
Undesirable - orange

- The highest reported success rate for bridge to transplant (92%) with HeartWare
- The most patient implants ≥5000 with the HeartMate II
- Fully magnetically suspended centrifugal pump with the Levacor

UNIQUE FEATURES OF THE JARVIK 2000 HEART

The Jarvik 2000 heart is about the size of a C battery and is implanted in the apex of the left ventricle, as shown in **Figs. 1** and **2**. Alternatively, it may be implanted as a biventricular assist system, which the authors call *total ventricular assist*, as shown in **Fig. 3**. **Fig. 4** shows the Jarvik 2000 and HeartMate II.

Figs. 5 and **6** show the tunneled abdominal cables typically used with VADs. The Jarvik 2000 also provides the option to use a percutaneous lead with power transmitted across the skin via a connector implanted behind the ear. This setup prevents trauma to the skin junction, because the connector is rigidly attached to the skull with bone screws, and because the scalp tissue is almost immobile. The scalp tissue is highly resistant to infection because it is so vascular and provides a high concentration of antibodies

and leucocytes to any head wound. The connector postcrossing the skin remains free of infection in 97% of cases up to 7.5 years. The advantages of delivering power to the pump this way are that no topical antibiotics are required, no wound dressing is needed, and the patient may bathe or shower normally, simply washing the connector with shampoo and drying the hair normally.

The Jarvik 2000 postauricular connector (**Fig. 7**) is the most successful long-term power access device used with any VAD. It. has

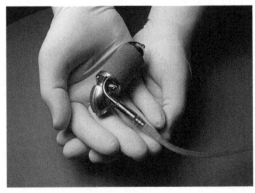

Fig. 1. The Jarvik 2000-C VAD.

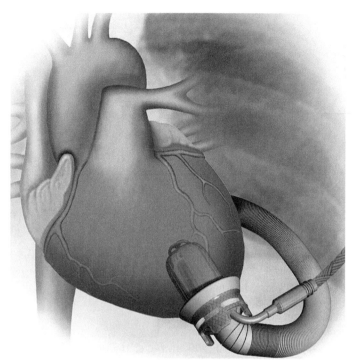

Fig. 2. The Jarvik 2000 implanted in the apex of the left ventricle, with the outflow graft anastomosed to the descending aorta.

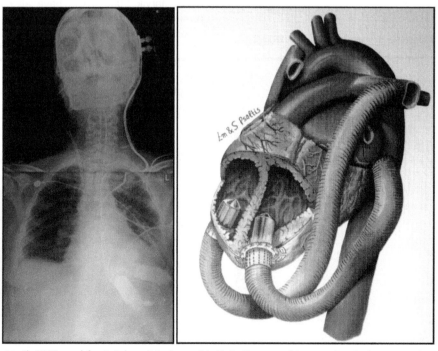

Fig. 3. The Jarvik 2000 used for total ventricular assist. Note the use of two postauricular connectors for power supply to the right and left pumps.

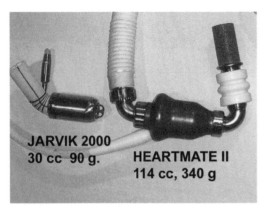

Fig. 4. The Jarvik 2000 and the HeartMate II. The HeartMate II inlet cannula (*upper right*) is approximately the size of the Jarvik 2000.

remained infection free for 7.5 years, has had no internal cable failure in more than 150 cases, and uses triple-redundant electrical conductors. If the external cable becomes damaged, patients can change it themselves, because the plug and receptacle are keyed to fit together only the correct way. Perhaps the greatest advantages of the postauricular connector are that it preserves a very normal body image, is cosmetically unnoticed in this age of cell phone cables worn on the ear, and does not interfere with clothing.

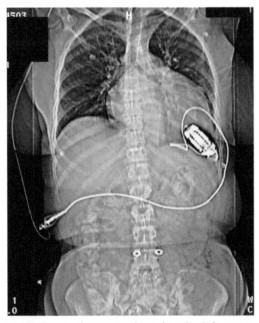

Fig. 5. The Jarvik 2000 implanted in the left ventricular apex.

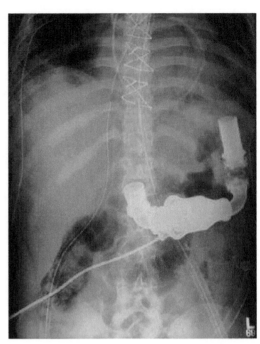

Fig. 6. The HeartMate II implanted in the abdomen.

RECENT IMPROVEMENT OF THE JARVIK 2000 BEARINGS

Blood-immersed bearings used with the Heart-Mate II, MicroMed DeBakey (MicroMed Cardiovascular, Inc., Houston, TX, USA), and the old model Jarvik 2000 VADs have all experienced formation of thrombus and associated serious adverse events. Usually the thrombus forms around the bearings in a crevice where the rotating bearing part is held by the stationary bearing part. This thrombus forms a thin fibrin band that completely surrounds the bearing, like a rope tied around a tree. The authors refer to this as

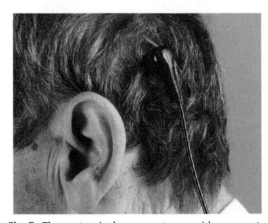

Fig. 7. The postauricular connector provides power to the Jarvik 2000.

ring thrombus. It cannot detach, and sometimes enlarges to become a thick ring of thrombus that may increase the friction on the pump, causing excessive motor power, or it may obstruct the flow path enough to diminish the blood flow or cause hemolysis. When the ring thrombus becomes large, portions of it can embolize.

The old design of the Jarvik 2000 used pin bearings illustrated in **Fig. 8**, and the current HeartWare II uses ball and cup bearings illustrated in **Fig. 9**. A crevice is present between the stationary bearing pin and the rotating bearing sleeve in the Jarvik 2000, and between the stationary cup and rotating ball in the HeartMate II. These crevices and similar crevices in other blood pump–bearing designs develop ring thrombus that is avoided with a new bearing design used in the Jarvik 2000, called cone bearings.

Fig. 10 shows the pin and sleeve–bearing design previously used in the Jarvik 2000.

The cone-bearing design used in the improved Jarvik 2000-C (**Fig. 11**) eliminates ring thrombus because no circumferential crevice is present in which ring thrombus can form. A rotating ceramic cone is supported by three ceramic blades. The blade tips have contours that match the shape of the cone surface. The spaces between the blades permit free, unobstructed flow for high washing, with no circumferential crevice in which thrombus can form a ring surrounding the rotor. The rotor (**Fig. 12**) is confined by three support blades at each end. This arrangement provides both radial-bearing support and thrust-bearing support. The rotor can spin freely but is confined and has practically no motion in the axial, tilt, or side-to-side directions. **Fig. 13** shows the way the bearing rings, which hold the bearing support blades, are nested into the housing. The rotor of the Jarvik 2000-C is shown in **Fig. 14**. The ceramic cone bearing components are the same on each end of the rotor (**Fig. 15**).

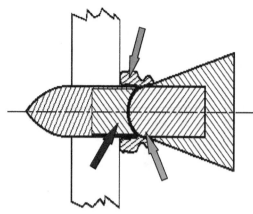

Fig. 9. The ball (*green arrow*) and cup (*purple arrow*) design presently used with the HeartMate II develops ring thrombus (*orange arrow*) beginning in the crevice surrounding the junction of the stationary and rotating surfaces.

The cone bearings are not hydrodynamic bearings. Blood-lubricated mixed-film lubrication is present where the stationary bearing support blade tips contact the rotating ceramic cones. As the bearing cone rotates, the boundary layer at its surface is drawn into the gap between the cone and the blade tips. Computational fluid dynamic modeling has shown a small pressure gradient between the upstream side and the downstream side of the blade (relative to the direction of rotation of the cone). The pressure gradient produced by the viscous surface drag of the cone on the blood washes the tiny gap between the blade tips and cones. The blades also act as wipers that would mechanically dislodge any material adhering to the cone surface, and this helps keep that surface completely free of thrombus (**Fig. 16**).

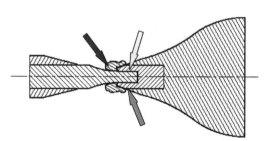

Fig. 8. The pin (*yellow arrow*) and sleeve (*blue arrow*)–bearing design is no longer used in the Jarvik 2000 because it developed ring thrombus (*red arrow*) in the crevice between the rotating and stationary surfaces.

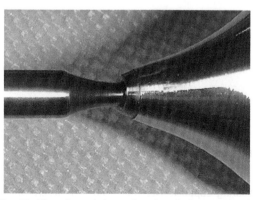

Fig. 10. The pin and sleeve–bearing design previously used in the Jarvik 2000.

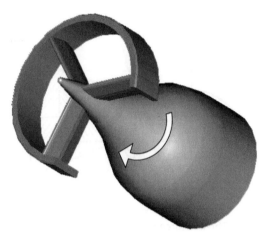

Fig. 11. The cone-bearing design used in the improved Jarvik 2000-C. This design eliminates ring thrombus because no circumferential crevice is present in which ring thrombus can form. A rotating ceramic cone (*gray*) is supported by three ceramic blades. The blade tips have contours that match the shape of the cone surface. The spaces between the blades permit free unobstructed flow for high washing.

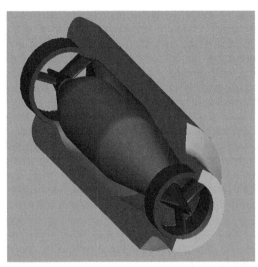

Fig. 13. The way the bearing rings, which hold the bearing support blades, are nested into the housing is illustrated. At each end of the pump the bearing rings are mounted flush with the housing, which forms a very clean junction with practically no crevice. This junction is very well washed by high flow, and no thrombus accumulates at this location.

IMPROVED INTERFACE BETWEEN THE JARVIK 2000 SURFACE AND THE APICAL MYOCARDIUM

The original model of the Jarvik 2000 used a smooth polished titanium housing in contact with the apical myocardial tissue, which forms the interface between the pump and the patient's heart. The junction between the outer surface of the blood pump and the myocardium formed

a crevice in which thrombus frequently formed, as shown in **Fig. 17**, which is a picture taken 3 years after implant when the patient received a donor heart. Although the patient had no thromboembolic events, and is currently in good health more than 9 years after implant of the Jarvik 2000, an adherent thrombus formed in the junction of the pump and the myocardium, and a ring thrombus approximately 3 mm in diameter formed at the inflow pin bearing.

The authors have modified the smooth outer surface of the original design to use a porous surface to prevent thrombus at the apex (**Fig. 18**). The cylindrical outer portion of the housing is now coated with a sintered microsphere surface, the

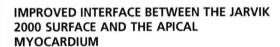

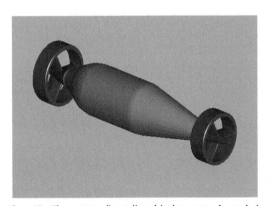

Fig. 12. The rotor (impeller blades not shown) is confined by three support blades at each end. This arrangement provides radial-bearing and thrust-bearing support. The rotor can spin freely but is confined and has practically no motion in the axial, tilt, or side-to-side directions.

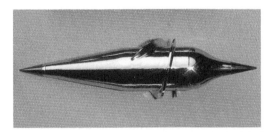

Fig. 14. The rotor of the Jarvik 2000-C with the black ceramic bearing cone on each end of the titanium rotor.

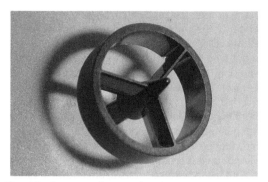

Fig. 15. The ceramic cone-bearing components are the same on each end of the rotor.

same as used with the lining of the HeartMate I or the inflow cannula of the HeartMate II. This surface was originally developed under an early National Institutes of Health research program in the late 1970s. The surface is thin enough that cellular ingrowth remains viable because of direct diffusion from the blood, and the surface often becomes endothelialized.

A well-integrated thrombus-free junction between the device and the patient's tissues is an essential element of any VAD that can be widely used for patients who are transplant candidates but who will most likely be supported permanently with the device.

The unique characteristics of the Jarvik 2000 are summarized in **Box 1**.

The data in **Fig. 19** illustrate the recent improvement of rotary VADs compared with the large pusher plate HeartMate I and other early designs. However, comparisons between the HeartMate II

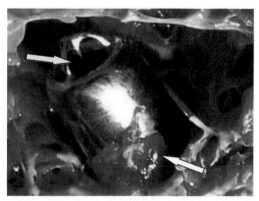

Fig. 17. An early Jarvik 2000 heart at 3 years after implant, removed when the patient underwent transplant. The white arrow shows a large thrombus in the crevice where the housing penetrates the myocardium at the apex. The yellow arrow indicates a small ring thrombus approximately 3 mm in diameter surrounding the inflow pin bearing.

and Jarvik 2000 are approximate because patient populations differed and the Jarvik 2000 was often used in patients judged too sick to have the HeartMate II with cardiopulmonary bypass. Jarvik 2000 cone-bearing cases exclude non–pump-related perioperative mortality. The green curve in **Fig. 19** shows the combined non–United States Jarvik 2000 pin-bearing pumps (both smooth and

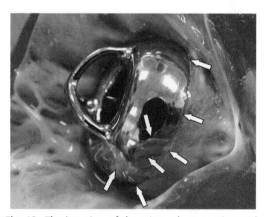

Fig. 18. The junction of the microsphere coating with the myocardial tissue at the apex is well healed by 2 months, and free of thrombus. A healthy adherent neointema is seen growing into the porous microsphere surface and stopping at the portion of the device that is smooth and polished. The white arrows indicate the junction of the smooth surface and the microsphere surface. What seems to be material on the smooth portion of the housing (*yellow arrows*) is a reflection of the endocardium and cut surface of the myocardium.

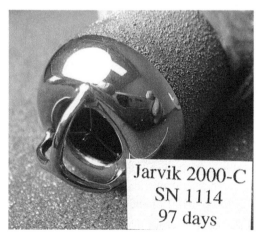

Fig. 16. A Jarvik 2000-C removed for transplant after 3 months with no thrombus present on the cone bearings.

Box 1
Unique characteristics of the Jarvik 2000

- Intraventricular placement with no pump pocket infection
- Safe if stopped in the event of accidental damage to external components
- Implanted off-bypass in most cases
- Postauricular connector gives superior reliability and quality of life for more than 7 years
- Very low incidence of cable infection
- High flex-life abdominal cable withstands greater than 50 million flex cycles
- Patients can adjust their own pump speed at home or away to meet the needs of exercise
- Intermittent low-speed controller prevents aortic valve deterioration
- Best fit for biventricular support; easy right/left balance

The randomized evaluation of mechanical assistance for the treatment of congestive heart failure (REMATCH)[6] control population, shown by the bright blue line in **Fig. 19**, had a dismal prognosis, with only 10% 2-year survival without mechanical support. Even with the HeartMate I, survival was only 22% at 2 years. Results with the earlier models of the Jarvik 2000 (pumps with pin bearings, with the smooth housing surface before the introduction of the microsphere coating, and without an important new control mode with intermittent low-speed controllers) are shown in green. Patient populations and indications for use differed between these patients and those in the HeartMate II DT study, shown in dark blue. Both results, showing 52% 2-year survival with the Jarvik 2000 and 58% 2-year survival with the HeartMate II, are more than double the survival rates with the HeartMate I. Additionally, the patients treated had a profile similar to that of the REMATCH controls. These findings certainly show marked improvement from the results with the large, noisy, and mechanically unreliable HeartMate I, and Novacor (WorldHeart Corporation).

The recent results with the HeartMate II bridge-to-transplant postmarket study are markedly improved, showing 90% survival at 6 months and 85% at 1 year. This tracks the heart transplant results. HeartWare has also reported results essentially the same as transplant, and a little higher than HeartMate II. But because no randomized

microsphere, abdominal cable and postauricular cable). The red curve gives the trend in the first 25 patients with the cone-bearing design. HeartMate II DT results are for the study randomized against HeartMate I. The HeartMate II results shown in orange are for the bridge-to-transplant postmarket study with no major device improvements.

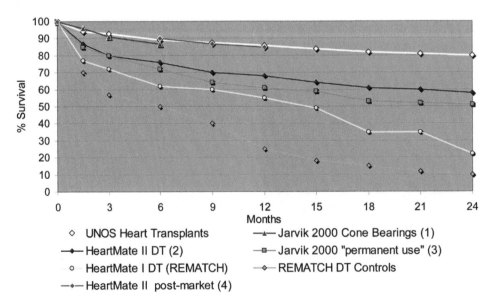

Fig. 19. Two-year survival with medical therapy alone, transplant, old and improved models of the Jarvik 2000, and old and improved models of HeartMate VADs. DT, destination therapy; REMATCH, randomized evaluation of mechanical assistance for the treatment of congestive heart failure.

studies have been performed, and because patient selection and the level of experience of the hospital teams treating the patients differ, the only reasonably conclusion possible is that VAD survival results are likely to equal transplant survival results, at least for 1 or 2 years. The initial Jarvik 2000 cone-bearing results also are showing a survival trend similar to that for transplant.

With these high survival rates, approval for payment by Medicare and most private insurance, and a high quality of life, VAD therapy is reaching the target of equaling transplant success.

SUMMARY

Major advances in VAD technology and the clinical acceptance of destination therapy for patients with contraindications to transplant raise the questions of what patient benefit is necessary to recommend VAD implant for long-term support in patients who are transplant candidates, and what are the appropriate indications for use and appropriate timing considerations for long-term VAD therapy in patients who qualify for transplant but are unlikely to obtain a donor.

The authors suggest that implantation for an indication of maintenance therapy, in which patients must wait at least 2 years while on the VAD before being listed with the United Network for Organ Sharing, would constitute an appropriate clinical avenue to study these issues. Despite whether this suggestion is implemented, the authors believe that clinical results are fast approaching the level of excellence achieved with transplant, and that widespread VAD use in patients for whom donor availability is insufficient is rapidly approaching.

REFERENCES

1. Alba AC, McDonald M, Rao V, et al. The effect of ventricular assist devices on long-term post-transplant outcomes: a systemic review of observational studies. Eur J Heart Fail 2011;13(7):785–95.
2. Slaughter MS, Rogers JG, Milano CA, et al. Advanced heart failure treated with continuous-flow left ventricular assist device. N Engl J Med 2009;361(23): 2241–51.
3. Stehllik J, Edwards LB, Kucheryavaya AY, et al. Registry of the International Society for Heart and Lung Transplantation: twenty-seventh official heart transplant report—2010. J Heart Lung Transplant 2010;29:1089–103.
4. Starling RC, Naka Y, Boyle AJ, et al. Results of the post-U.S. Food and Drug Administration approval study with a continuous flow left ventricular assist device as a bridge to heart transplantation. J Am Coll Cardiol 2010;57:1890–8.
5. INTERMACS Interagency Registry for Mechanically Assisted Circulatory Support: Quarterly Statistical Report. Implant dates: March 1, 2006–June 30, 2010. Available at: http://www.uab.edu/ctsresearch/intermacs/Document%20Library/INTERMACS%20Federal%20Partners%20Quarterly%20Report%20June%202009%20website.pdf. Accessed August 13, 2011.
6. Rose EA, Gellins AC, Moskowitz AJ, et al. Long-term use of a left ventricular assist device for end-stage heart failure. N Engl J Med 2001;345:1435–43.

Editorial Comments on "VAD or Transplant"

John A. Elefteriades, MD

KEY CONCEPTS

In his article titled "VAD or Transplant?" Dr Robert Jarvik, the brilliant motivating force behind artificial heart technology for nearly half a century, challenges us to consider which we want, a transplant or a ventricular assist device (VAD). He points out that the presumed superiority of transplant, in survival and quality of life, is narrowing or, perhaps, even reversing as VAD technology advances.

STRENGTHS

To see the competition between VAD and transplant through Dr Jarvik's eyes is a true eye opener.

It makes the reader wonder whether transplant really is better. Which would one of us choose if we had advanced heart failure? The editors might opt for a VAD.

WEAKNESSES

Dr Jarvik is understandably partial to the Jarvik 2000 device, but the authors also are very fond of this VAD, which is relatively noninvasive to place and simple to operate. It is premature to claim final victory for VAD over transplant, however, because VAD technology has many serious obstacles to overcome, most notably, stroke, hemorrhage, and infection.

Section of Cardiac Surgery, Yale University School of Medicine, Boardman 2, 333 Cedar Street, New Haven, CT 06510, USA
E-mail address: john.elefteriades@yale.edu

Cardiol Clin 29 (2011) 597
doi:10.1016/j.ccl.2011.07.008

Who Needs an RVAD in Addition to an LVAD?

David J. Kaczorowski, MD, Y. Joseph Woo, MD*

KEYWORDS
- Heart failure • Ventricular assist devices
- Mechanical circulatory support • Right ventricular failure

Congestive heart failure is a major health problem. It is increasing in prevalence and is associated with a high mortality.[1,2] Although heart transplantation remains the gold standard for treatment of end-stage heart failure, hearts suitable for donation are scarce. Given the lack of hearts available for transplantation, other modes of therapy for managing end-stage heart failure are necessary. Mechanical circulatory support has become an accepted modality for the treatment of end-stage heart failure. Mechanical circulatory support devices (MCSDs) can be used as a bridge to transplantation with the intent of supporting the failing heart until transplantation. Alternatively, MCSDs can be used as destination therapy whereby the device is implanted as a permanent method of supporting the heart.

Data has demonstrated that the use of left ventricular assist devices (LVAD) for the management of end-stage heart failure results in superior outcomes when compared with medical management.[3,4] Furthermore, the technology used in the engineering of these devices continues to improve. Devices are becoming progressively smaller, and novel energy transmission systems are being developed. Despite both clinical and technological progress, obstacles to the successful use of mechanical circulatory support for the management of heart failure still exist. Right ventricular (RV) failure in the setting of LVAD insertion is one such problem.

RV DYSFUNCTION NEGATIVELY IMPACTS OUTCOMES AFTER LVAD INSERTION

The presence or absence of RV dysfunction is a critical determinant of outcomes in patients undergoing MCSD placement. Analysis of international registry data has identified several risk factors for early mortality after ventricular assist device placement, including advanced age, thrombocytopenia, leukocytosis, diabetes, ventilator dependence, renal dysfunction, and concurrent placement of a rent ventricular assist device (RVAD). Of all of these, RV dysfunction requiring biventricular support was identified as the most prominent risk factor for early mortality in patients undergoing ventricular assist device placement.[5]

Several other studies have documented poorer outcomes in patients with significant RV dysfunction that undergo LVAD placement. Dang and colleagues[6] examined outcomes of 108 patients with chronic congestive heart failure who underwent LVAD implantation at a single center. Of these, 42 patients experienced RV dysfunction and 14 ultimately underwent RVAD insertion. The investigators found that patients with right heart failure requiring intravenous inotropes, pulmonary vasodilators, or subsequent RVAD insertion for RV support had significantly worse outcomes. Specifically, higher rates of renal failure, higher rates of reoperation, greater length of intensive-care-unit stay, and higher early mortality were observed in patients with RV dysfunction compared with those that did not have RV dysfunction. Furthermore, of the patients that required RVAD placement after LVAD insertion, only 35.7% could be bridged to transplantation compared with 89.9% of the patients undergoing LVAD insertion without evidence of postoperative RV dysfunction.[6]

Farrar and coinvestigators[7] analyzed data on 213 patients from 35 hospitals who underwent

The authors have nothing to disclose.

Division of Cardiovascular Surgery, University of Pennsylvania, 3400 Spruce Street, 6 Silverstein Pavilion, Philadelphia, PA 19104, USA

* Corresponding author.

E-mail address: joseph.woo@uphs.upenn.edu

Cardiol Clin 29 (2011) 599–605

doi:10.1016/j.ccl.2011.08.011

ventricular assist device placement. Of these patients, 74 underwent LVAD insertion and 139 underwent biventricular assist device (BiVAD) placement. There were several statistically significant differences between the groups preoperatively. The patients that required BiVAD placement were found to have a lower preoperative cardiac index, higher creatinine, higher bilirubin, and higher frequency of mechanical ventilation compared with those undergoing LVAD placement. Although the group of patients that underwent BiVAD placement was clearly afflicted with more severe illness preoperatively, it is notable that 89% of the patients that underwent LVAD placement survived to transplantation, whereas only 58% of the patients that underwent BiVAD placement survived to ultimately undergo transplantation.[7]

In a retrospective analysis, Kormos and colleagues[8] examined preoperative data and the clinical course of 40 patients that underwent LVAD placement. Of these patients, 31 patients had RV failure, defined as a RV ejection fraction (RVEF) less than 20%. The group of patients that had RV failure was further subclassified based on the ease of clinical management of the RV dysfunction. Fourteen patients required only short-term (defined as less than 7 days) inotropic support. Seven patients required a greater degree of inotropic support, and 10 other patients required placement of an RVAD after initial LVAD placement. Of the 14 that required only short-term inotropic support for the RV, 100% successfully underwent heart transplantation and were subsequently discharged from the hospital. In contrast, only 5 of 7 patients (71%) in the group requiring more prolonged inotropic support for the RV survived to undergo transplantation. Furthermore, only 4 of 10 patients (40%) that required RVAD placement survived to transplantation.[8]

EARLY PLANNED RV SUPPORT CAN ALLEVIATE ADVERSE CONSEQUENCES OF RV DYSFUNCTION

It is clear that RV dysfunction can negatively influence outcomes after LVAD placement. Recent data is also emerging that demonstrates that early planned RVAD placement can mitigate adverse effects of RV dysfunction. Magliato and coinvestigators[9] examined outcomes of 19 patients in heart failure that was unresponsive to medical therapy who underwent planned BiVAD placement as a bridge to transplantation. In this study, all patients were in cardiogenic shock before BiVAD placement and 3 patients were actually receiving cardiopulmonary resuscitation before implantation of the devices. The severity of illness of this cohort

of patients is further highlighted by the preoperative characteristics of this group. In this group of patients, 68% were receiving mechanical ventilation, an intra-aortic balloon pump (IABP) was present in 89%, 3 or more inotropes were being used in 84%, hyperbilirubinemia was present in 59%, and acute renal failure was present in 63%. Despite the degree of illness in this cohort of patients, 59% of patients were successfully bridged to transplantation and 90% of those patients survived posttransplantation.[9]

In another study, Tsukui and colleagues[10] performed a retrospective analysis of 73 patients that underwent BiVAD placement at a single center. Before the implantation of the devices, all patients were on 1 or more inotropic agents and 77% of patients had an IABP. In this group of patients, the overall survival was 69%. Of the surviving patients, 42 patients (84%) underwent transplant, 5 patients (10%) were weaned from mechanical circulatory support, and 3 patients (6%) remained supported by BiVADs.

The studies by Tsukui and Magliato demonstrate that planned institution of biventricular support using BiVADs can result in good outcomes, even in severely ill patients. With these findings in mind, outcomes of 266 patients undergoing LAVD or BiVAD placement at the authors' center over a 12-year period between 1995 and 2007 were retrospectively analyzed.[11] Of these 266 patients, 167 (63%) underwent LVAD placement alone and 99 (37%) underwent BiVAD placement. To address whether early planned BiVAD placement resulted in improved outcomes compared with delayed BiVAD placement, the group of patients that underwent BiVAD placement was further subdivided based on the timing of RVAD insertion. Seventy-one patients underwent planned BiVAD placement. This group included only patients whereby the plan to place an RVAD was predetermined before taking the patients to the operating room. Twenty-eight patients first underwent LVAD placement followed by subsequent RVAD placement. In this subgroup of patients, the median time to RVAD insertion was 2 days. Preoperative characteristics of the planned and delayed RVAD subgroups were similar.

As expected, superior survival to transplantation, survival to hospital discharge, and long-term survival were observed in the group of patients that underwent LVAD insertion alone compared with the other groups. Of note, survival to hospital discharge was also significantly better in the group of patients that underwent planned RVAD placement (51%) compared with the group that underwent delayed RVAD placement (29%). In addition, both 1-year and long-term survival were also better in the planned RVAD group compared with the delayed RVAD group. Furthermore, there was a trend toward improved survival to transplantation in patients that underwent planned RVAD insertion compared with those undergoing delayed RVAD insertion.[11] These findings demonstrate that early planned institution of RV support can result in superior outcomes when compared with delayed RVAD placement.

PREDICTORS OF RV DYSFUNCTION NECESSITATING MECHANICAL SUPPORT IN PATIENTS UNDERGOING LVAD PLACEMENT

Currently, with the exception of the sporadic use of implantable ventricular assist devices, such as the Thoratec Heartmate 2 (Thoratec, Pleasanton, CA, USA) and the Heartware ventricular assist device (HVAD, HeartWare International, Framingham, MA, USA), as both right and left heart support, destination therapy is essentially only possible for patients with isolated left ventricular failure.[12–15] Furthermore, early planned institution of RV mechanical support can result in superior outcomes compared with delayed RVAD insertion in appropriately selected patients. For these reasons, predicting which patients will require mechanical support for RV failure in the setting of LVAD placement is critical.

Several risk factors for RV dysfunction after LVAD placement have been identified (**Box 1**). In their retrospective analysis of 108 patients with chronic congestive heart failure that underwent LVAD placement at a single center, Dang and colleagues[6] sought out risk factors for right heart failure. Of the variables examined in their study, only elevated intraoperative central venous pressure (CVP) was found to be a significant predictor of right heart failure after LVAD insertion with an odds ratio (OR) of 1.187.

In another retrospective analysis with specific focus on RV dysfunction, Kavarana and coinvestigators reviewed data on 69 patients that underwent LVAD insertion.[16] In this series, RV dysfunction was defined as the need for inotropic support for 14 or more days or the need for RVAD insertion. Of the 69 patients that underwent LVAD placement, 21 (30.4%) experienced RV dysfunction and only 1 of these patients underwent RVAD insertion. Although the baseline characteristics, including age, sex, cause of heart failure, and duration of support, were similar among groups, patients who developed RV dysfunction were noted to have a significantly higher preoperative bilirubin, with a trend toward higher aspartate aminotransferase (AST) levels and serum creatinine levels. Although it did not reach statistical significance, lower preoperative RV

Box 1
Parameters identified as risk factors for RV failure after LVAD placement

Several risk factors for RV failure after LVAD insertion have been identified and are listed here:

Clinical

> Severe preoperative RV dysfunction
>
> Previous cardiac surgery
>
> Need for preoperative mechanical ventilation
>
> Need for preoperative mechanical circulatory support
>
> Female sex
>
> Smaller body size
>
> Nonischemic cause of heart failure

Hemodynamic

> Low cardiac index
>
> Elevated CVP
>
> Low systolic blood pressure
>
> Low RV stroke work and RV stroke work index
>
> Low pulmonary artery pressure

Laboratory

> Elevated blood urea nitrogen, creatinine
>
> Elevated bilirubin, aspartate aminotransferase, alanine aminotransferase

Echocardiographic

> Grade III/IV tricuspid insufficiency
>
> RV short/long axis ratio greater than 0.6
>
> Low tricuspid annular motion

---

stroke work index (RVSWI) was observed in the group that experienced RV dysfunction.

Santambrogio and colleagues[17] examined data on 48 patients who underwent LVAD placement. In this study, RV failure occurred in 16% of the patients. The investigators compared preoperative data on patients that developed RV failure with data on those that did not develop RV failure to help identify risk factors for RV failure. They found a greater frequency of mechanical ventilation in the patients that developed RV failure (25.0%) compared with those that did not (5.1%). In addition, patients that ultimately developed RV failure had higher serum levels of blood urea nitrogen (BUN), creatinine, AST, and alanine aminotransferase but not bilirubin. A multivariate analysis was not performed in this study.[17]

To identify preoperative risk factors for RV failure in another study, preoperative characteristics and hemodynamic data was analyzed in 100 patients undergoing LVAD placement at a single center.[18] RV device placement was required in 11 patients. The investigators found that RVAD insertion was more common in female patients, younger patients, smaller patients, and patients with myocarditis. The mean PA pressure and RVSWI were both significantly lower in the group of patients that required RVAD placement when compared with those that did not.[18]

To further elucidate preoperative risk factors for RV failure, investigators from the same center analyzed data from 245 patients that underwent LVAD placement between 1991 and 2001.[19] RVAD placement was required in 23 patients (9%) after LVAD insertion. Preoperative clinical and hemodynamic data on patients that required RVAD placement and those that did not was compared. Female sex, small body surface area, nonischemic cause, preoperative mechanical ventilation, circulatory support before LVAD insertion, low mean and diastolic PA pressures, low RV stroke work (RVSW), and low RVSWI were identified as risk factors in a univariate analysis. In a multivariate analysis, only preoperative circulatory support (OR 5.3), female sex (OR 4.5) and non-ischemic cause (OR 3.3) were identified as risk factors for RV failure. Of note, RVSW and RVSWI were not tested in the multivariate model because data was missing for a large portion of the patients.[19]

In a larger and more recent report, Kormos and coinvestigators[20] studied 484 patients enrolled in the HeartMate II left ventricular assist device bridge-to-transplantation trial; data was compared between patients with and without RV failure. In this study, 30 patients (6%) underwent RVAD placement, 35 patients (7%) required inotropes for 14 days or longer to support the RV, and 33 patients (7%) required late use of inotropes for RV support. A multivariate analysis was performed, and several risk factors for RV failure were identified. Need for preoperative ventilator support (OR 5.5), central venous pressure/pulmonary capillary wedge pressure ratio of greater than 0.63 (OR 2.3), and BUN greater than 39 mg/dL (OR 2.1) were found to be statistically significant, independent predictors of RV failure.[20]

Although these studies have focused on clinical characteristics, including hemodynamic measurements and laboratory values, others have focused on echocardiographic parameters as potential predictors of RV failure after LVAD insertion. Potapov and coinvestigators[21] retrospectively analyzed echocardiographic data on 54 patients that underwent LVAD placement. Nine patients experienced RV failure defined by RVAD placement or the presence of 2 of several clinical criteria, including mean arterial pressure less than 55 mm Hg, CVP greater than 16 mm Hg, mixed venous saturation less than 55%, cardiac index (CI) less than 2 L/min/m^2, or high-dose inotropic support, all in the absence of cardiac tamponade. The echocardiographic parameters studied included tricuspid valve incompetence, RV end-diastolic diameter, RVEF, right atrial dimension, and short/long axis ratio of the RV. The investigators found that when the RV short/long axis ratio was less than 0.6, RV failure occurred in 7% of the patients. In contrast, RV failure occurred in 50% of patients with a short/long axis greater than or equal to 0.6. This finding reached statistical significance in a multivariate analysis with an OR of 4.4. In addition, 75% of the patients with grade III or IV tricuspid insufficiency (TI) developed right heart failure, whereas only 12% of the patients with grade I or II TI developed right heart failure. Grade III or IV TI was also found to be statistically significant in a multivariate analysis of predictors of RV failure with an OR of 4.7.[21]

Seeking to identify predictors of right heart failure after LVAD placement, Puwanant and associates[22] examined several preoperative echocardiographic parameters in 33 patients that underwent LVAD insertion. In this study, 11 patients (33%) experienced RV failure (as defined by a need for inotropic agents or pulmonary vasodilators for 14 days or longer) and 2 of these patients required placement of an RVAD. Preoperative parameters that were examined included RV fractional area of change, tricuspid annular motion, right atrial volume index, RV index of myocardial performance, hepatic vein Doppler velocities, tricuspid regurgitation severity, and RV systolic pressures. Significantly lower tricuspid annular motion was observed in patients with RV failure after LVAD insertion. This finding held true in the presence of significant tricuspid regurgitation. The investigators found that tricuspid annular motion less than 7.5 mm predicts RV failure after LVAD placement with a specificity of 91%.[22]

QUANTITATIVE SCORING SYSTEMS FOR PREDICTING THE NEED FOR RV SUPPORT

Given the serious consequences of RV failure after LVAD placement, identifying patients who will benefit from RVAD placement is critical. Although several discreet risk factors for RV failure after LVAD placement were identified by the studies previously described, none of them provide an algorithm for quantitative assessment of an individual patient's risk for the need for RV support. To develop a scoring system that can help identify which patients undergoing LVAD insertion will require an RVAD, data from 266 patients who underwent LVAD placement at the authors' institution between 1995 and 2007 were reviewed in a retrospective manner.[23] Of the 266 patients in this study, 167 (63%) underwent isolated LVAD placement only and 99 (37%) required RVAD insertion. A broad range of device types were used in these patients.

Immediate preoperative clinical, hemodynamic, and laboratory data were analyzed. A multivariate logistic regression analysis was performed, and several variables that predicted the need for RV mechanical assistance were identified. Several of these values were hemodynamic parameters, including a CI less than 2.2 L/min/m^2, RVSWI less than or equal to 0.25 mm Hg L/m^2, and systolic blood pressure less than or equal to 96 mm Hg. Creatinine greater than or equal to 1.9 mg/dL was the only laboratory value found to be of statistical significance in the multivariate regression analysis. Two clinical parameters, severe RV dysfunction before ventricular assist device placement and previous cardiac surgery, were also found to be significant in the multivariate analysis.[23]

These 6 independent parameters were then assigned a coefficient weighted by the OR determined in the multivariate logistic regression analysis. An equation was then created that represented the sum of the weighted variables as follows: 18 (CI) + 18 (RVSWI) + 17 (creatinine) + 16 (previous cardiac surgery) + 16 (severe preoperative RV dysfunction) +13 systolic blood pressure. If the patient has the identified risk factor, a score of 1 is placed into the equation for that variable. If the patient does not possess a particular risk factor, a score of 0 is placed into the equation for that variable. For example, if a patient has a CI of 1.4 L/min/m^2, then a value of 1 would be placed in the equation for the value CI. Conversely, if the index was 3.0 L/min/m^2, then a value of 0 would be entered. The maximal possible score is 98. Using a threshold value of 50 and applying the scoring system to the cohort studied revealed that the equation had a sensitivity of 83% and a specificity of 80%. Furthermore, 96% of the patients with scores less than 30 underwent successful LVAD insertion without the need for mechanical support of the RV, whereas 89% of patients with scores greater than or equal to 65 required RV support.[23] This scoring system is derived from single-center data and will require prospective evaluation, but it may serve as an extremely valuable tool for identifying patients that require biventricular mechanical support.

To also help identify patients that might develop RV failure in the setting of LVAD insertion, Matthews and coinvestigators[24] retrospectively evaluated clinical, echocardiographic, hemodynamic, and laboratory data on 197 patients undergoing LVAD placement at their center. In this study, RV failure was defined as the use of inotropic support for greater than 14 days, use of inhaled nitric oxide for greater than 48 hours postoperatively, discharge from the hospital on an inotropic agent, or right-sided mechanical circulatory support of any kind (either extracorporeal membrane oxygenation or RVAD). According to this definition, 68 patients (35%) experienced RV dysfunction in this study. Of these patients, 29 received mechanical RV support.[24]

A multivariate analysis was performed. Several variables, including need for vasopressor support, AST greater than 80 IU/L, bilirubin greater than 2.0 mg/dL, creatinine greater than 2.3 mg/dL, or the need for renal replacement therapy, were identified as independent predictors of RV failure. Point values were then assigned to each of these variables based on the calculated OR. A vasopressor requirement was assigned 4 points, elevated creatinine was assigned 3 points, elevated bilirubin was assigned 2.5 points, and elevated AST was assigned 2 points. The RV failure score is then calculated as the sum of points awarded for each of the variables that are present. The investigators found that when applied to their cohort, patients with a score of greater than 5.5 had a 15-fold greater risk of developing RV failure than those with a score less than 3.0 and also a 3-fold greater risk compared with those with a score between 3.0 and 5.0. Although a score greater than or equal to 5.5 yielded a positive predictive value of 80%, the sensitivity was found to be only 35%. The investigators found that this scoring system performed significantly better as a predictor of RV failure than several other individual parameters, including severe RV failure on echocardiography, RVSWI, pulmonary vascular resistance, transpulmonary gradient, pulmonary artery systolic pressure, or right atrial pressure.[24]

The studies by Matthews and Fitzpatrick[23,24] represent efforts to quantitate the risk for RV failure after LVAD insertion. Although both studies identified elevated creatinine as risk factor for RV failure, the variables that factor into the equations developed in each of these studies are otherwise different. Each of these studies was based on experiences at individual centers and this may be one factor that led to these differences. More importantly, the study by Fitzpatrick and colleagues[23] focused on patients requiring mechanical assistance for RV support. In contrast, in the study by Matthews and coinvestigators,[24] the definition used for RV dysfunction was much broader and included patients who received inotropic support for greater than 14 days, inhaled nitric oxide for greater than 48 hours postoperatively, or were discharged from the hospital on an inotropic agent, in addition to patients who received RV mechanical circulatory support. Despite these differences, these scoring systems may assist in clinical decision making when considering the risk of RV dysfunction or the need for RV mechanical circulatory support after LVAD placement.

SUMMARY

Ventricular assist device insertion has become an important mode of therapy for end-stage heart failure. Currently, LVADs can be used both to bridge patients to transplant and as destination therapy. RV dysfunction is an important source of morbidity and mortality after LVAD insertion. Recent data demonstrates that early planned institution of RV support can mitigate the potential adverse consequences of RV dysfunction after LVAD placement. Although identifying which patients will require mechanical support for the RV is imperative, it remains challenging. Several studies have identified individual clinical, laboratory, hemodynamic, and echocardiographic parameters that may serve as risk factors for RV dysfunction after LVAD placement. Furthermore, scoring systems have been established to help quantitatively predict the potential need for RV support after LVAD placement. In addition to clinical judgment, these quantitative scoring systems may serve as useful tools in the identification of patients that may require mechanical support for the RV.

REFERENCES

1. McMurray JJ. Clinical practice. Systolic heart failure. N Engl J Med 2010;362(3):228–38.
2. Jessup M, Brozena S. Heart failure. N Engl J Med 2003;348(20):2007–18.
3. Rose EA, Gelijns AC, Moskowitz AJ, et al. Long-term use of a left ventricular assist device for end-stage heart failure. N Engl J Med 2001;345(20):1435–43.
4. Slaughter MS, Rogers JG, Milano CA, et al. Advanced heart failure treated with continuous-flow left ventricular assist device. N Engl J Med 2009; 361(23):2241–51.
5. Deng MC, Edwards LB, Hertz MI, et al. Mechanical circulatory support device database of the International Society for Heart and Lung Transplantation: third annual report–2005. J Heart Lung Transplant 2005;24(9):1182–7.
6. Dang NC, Topkara VK, Mercando M, et al. Right heart failure after left ventricular assist device implantation in patients with chronic congestive heart failure. J Heart Lung Transplant 2006; 25(1):1–6.
7. Farrar DJ, Hill JD, Pennington DG, et al. Preoperative and postoperative comparison of patients with univentricular and biventricular support with the Thoratec ventricular assist device as a bridge to cardiac transplantation. J Thorac Cardiovasc Surg 1997;113(1):202–9.
8. Kormos RL, Gasior TA, Kawai A, et al. Transplant candidate's clinical status rather than right ventricular function defines need for univentricular versus biventricular support. J Thorac Cardiovasc Surg 1996;111(4):773–82.
9. Magliato KE, Kleisli T, Soukiasian HJ, et al. Biventricular support in patients with profound cardiogenic shock: a single center experience. ASAIO J 2003; 49(4):475–9.
10. Tsukui H, Teuteberg JJ, Murali S, et al. Biventricular assist device utilization for patients with morbid congestive heart failure: a justifiable strategy. Circulation 2005;112(9 Suppl):I65–72.
11. Fitzpatrick JR III, Frederick JR, Hiesinger W, et al. Early planned institution of biventricular mechanical circulatory support results in improved outcomes compared with delayed conversion of a left ventricular assist device to a biventricular assist device. J Thorac Cardiovasc Surg 2009; 137(4):971–7.
12. Strueber M, Meyer AL, Malehsa D, et al. Successful use of the HeartWare HVAD rotary blood pump for biventricular support. J Thorac Cardiovasc Surg 2010;140(4):936–7.
13. Hetzer R, Krabatsch T, Stepanenko A, et al. Long-term biventricular support with the HeartWare implantable continuous flow pump. J Heart Lung Transplant 2010;29(7):822–4.
14. Loebe M, Bruckner B, Reardon MJ, et al. Initial clinical experience of total cardiac replacement with dual HeartMate-II axial flow pumps for severe biventricular heart failure. Methodist Debakey Cardiovasc J 2011;7(1):40–4.
15. Loforte A, Monica PL, Montalto A, et al. HeartWare third-generation implantable continuous flow pump as biventricular support: mid-term follow-up. Interact Cardiovasc Thorac Surg 2011;12(3):458–60.
16. Kavarana MN, Pessin-Minsley MS, Urtecho J, et al. Right ventricular dysfunction and organ failure in left ventricular assist device recipients: a continuing problem. Ann Thorac Surg 2002;73(3):745–50.
17. Santambrogio L, Bianchi T, Fuardo M, et al. Right ventricular failure after left ventricular assist device insertion: preoperative risk factors. Interact Cardiovasc Thorac Surg 2006;5(4):379–82.
18. Fukamachi K, McCarthy PM, Smedira NG, et al. Preoperative risk factors for right ventricular failure after implantable left ventricular assist device insertion. Ann Thorac Surg 1999;68(6):2181–4.

19. Ochiai Y, McCarthy PM, Smedira NG, et al. Predictors of severe right ventricular failure after implantable left ventricular assist device insertion: analysis of 245 patients. Circulation 2002;106(12 Suppl 1):I198–202.

20. Kormos RL, Teuteberg JJ, Pagani FD, et al. Right ventricular failure in patients with the HeartMate II continuous-flow left ventricular assist device: incidence, risk factors, and effect on outcomes. J Thorac Cardiovasc Surg 2010;139(5):1316–24.

21. Potapov EV, Stepanenko A, Dandel M, et al. Tricuspid incompetence and geometry of the right ventricle as predictors of right ventricular function after implantation of a left ventricular assist device. J Heart Lung Transplant 2008;27(12):1275–81.

22. Puwanant S, Hamilton KK, Klodell CT, et al. Tricuspid annular motion as a predictor of severe right ventricular failure after left ventricular assist device implantation. J Heart Lung Transplant 2008;27(10):1102–7.

23. Fitzpatrick JR III, Frederick JR, Hsu VM, et al. Risk score derived from pre-operative data analysis predicts the need for biventricular mechanical circulatory support. J Heart Lung Transplant 2008;27(12):1286–92.

24. Matthews JC, Koelling TM, Pagani FD, et al. The right ventricular failure risk score a pre-operative tool for assessing the risk of right ventricular failure in left ventricular assist device candidates. J Am Coll Cardiol 2008;51(22):2163–72.

Editorial Comments on "Who Needs an RVAD in Addition to an LVAD?"

John A. Elefteriades, MD

KEY CONCEPTS

Drs David J. Kaczorowski and Y. Joseph Woo, authors of "Who Needs an RVAD in Addition to an LVAD?" make the very important point that late, second-thought, right ventricular assist device (RVAD) placement leads to poorer survival compared with a priori placement during the same operation as left ventricular assist device (LVAD) placement. The investigators thoroughly review the pertinent literature. They identify 2 numerical grading systems for RVAD decision making.

STRENGTHS

Most useful is Table 1, which identifies clinical (severe antecedent right ventricular [RV] dysfunction, prior cardiac surgery, mechanical ventilation, intra-aortic balloon pump, female sex, small body size, ischemic cardiomyopathy), hemodynamic (low cardiac index, high central venous pressure, low blood pressure, low RV stroke work or RV stroke work index, low pulmonary artery pressure), laboratory (high serum urea nitrogen, high creatinine, and high hepatocellular enzyme levels), and echocardiographic (III/IV + tricuspid regurgitation, dilated RV, low tricuspid annular motion) predictors for RV failure after LVAD placement.

WEAKNESSES

The studies of the RVAD issue are disparate (definition of RV failure, devices used, end points) and hard to assimilate into a unified whole with consistent findings and recommendations. There is no question that a patient who needs an RVAD really needs it and needs it sooner rather than later, but, on the other hand, an RVAD complicates the operation and the aftercare, first and foremost because the RVAD will be external, requiring the blood to exit the patient. The final on this issue will not be in for some time. Technology may advance to the point that RV support is easily feasible and internal.

Section of Cardiac Surgery, Yale University School of Medicine, Boardman 2, 333 Cedar Street, New Haven, CT 06510, USA
E-mail address: john.elefteriades@yale.edu

Cardiol Clin 29 (2011) 607
doi:10.1016/j.ccl.2011.07.001
0733-8651/11/$ – see front matter © 2011 Published by Elsevier Inc

Toward Total Implantability Using Free-Range Resonant Electrical Energy Delivery System: Achieving Untethered Ventricular Assist Device Operation Over Large Distances

Benjamin Waters, BS[a], Alanson Sample, PhD[a],
Joshua Smith, PhD[a,b], Pramod Bonde, MD[c],*

KEYWORDS

- Free-Range Resonant Electrical Energy Delivery system
- Ventricular assist device • Heart disease • Heart failure
- Wireless power • Mechanical support

THE PROBLEM

Heart failure is a terminal disease with a very poor prognosis and constitutes Medicare's greatest area of spending, with annual expenditures close to \$35 billion.[1] The gold standard of treatment for this disease remains heart transplant; however, only a minority (approximately 2000 per year) of patients can benefit from transplants because of continuing donor shortage.

Another alternative, which has shown promise, is mechanical circulatory assistance with ventricular assist devices (VAD).[1] An estimated 100,000 patients worldwide can benefit from VAD therapy.[1] The benefit of VAD technology was demonstrated by the randomized evaluation of mechanical assistance for the treatment of congestive heart failure trial, which showed a 50% survival benefit for patients assigned to the VAD arm compared with those undergoing maximal medical management.[2] The same trial, however, also showed the limitations with the first-generation VADs in terms of large size and mechanical failure.[2–4] These findings prompted researchers and industry to concentrate their efforts in minimizing the size of the device, which has been achieved in the past decade with miniature axial and centrifugal pump technology. This advancement has allowed the use of these devices in smaller patients, who were not candidates in the past.[5]

[a] Department of Electrical Engineering, University of Washington, Box 352350,185 Stevens Way, Seattle, WA 98195-2350, USA
[b] Department of Computer Science and Engineering, University of Washington, Box 352350,185 Stevens Way, Seattle, WA 98195-2350, USA
[c] Section of Cardiac Surgery, Yale School of Medicine, 330 Cedar Street, Boardman 204, New Haven, CT 06520, USA
* Corresponding author.
E-mail address: prambond@hotmail.com

Cardiol Clin 29 (2011) 609–625
doi:10.1016/j.ccl.2011.08.002
0733-8651/11/\$ – see front matter © 2011 Elsevier Inc. All rights reserved.

Table 1
Distribution of ESIs among various risk categories

Variable	Non-ESI %	ESI %	P Value
Before 2000	55	45	P<.001
After 2000	80	20	
Nonobese	78	22	P<.03
Obese	65	35	
Cannula	69	31	P = .03
Driveline	78	22	
LVAD	77	23	P = .09
BiVAD	67	33	
Continuous	82	18	P = .17
Pulsatile	75	25	
Elective	81	19	P = .42
Nonelective	72	28	

Abbreviations: BiVAD, biventricular assist device; LVAD, left ventricular assist device.

A highly conservative approach is still practiced when offering VAD therapy to end-stage heart failure patients because of the associated adverse events, predominantly including the occurrence of repeated infections.[6] Infections occur despite the improved technology that typifies the smaller, durable designs with a single moving part that were introduced in the past decade.

Full advantage of these improvements is not realized because of essentially unchanged peripherals, including the percutaneous driveline for data retrieval and power supply.

A relationship among exit site infections (ESIs), pump pocket infection, and subsequent sepsis has been clearly shown. ESIs are influenced by constant exposure to the outside environment. Patients receiving VADs experience repeated infections, necessitating multiple antibiotics and repeated hospitalizations for surgical debridements. Infection also poses a therapeutic dilemma in terms of ever-increasing resistant colonization. ESIs often lead to subsequent pump infections, causing episodic bacteremia.[7–11]

Compared with other metallic implants (eg, cardiovascular implants, <2%; prosthetic valve endocarditis, 2%–4%[12,13]; orthopedic implants, such as hip and knee arthroplasty, <1%[14]), VADs pose a prohibitively high rate of infection, with reported incidence reaching 70% at the end of 1 year.[1–11,15–18]

VADs differ uniquely from other metallic implants because of the presence of a percutaneous drive line communicating with the exterior environment. As advancements move toward even longer durations of support on VADs,[4,5] the risk of ESIs continues to increase temporally, hampering quality of life and leading to repeated hospitalizations for antibiotic treatment or surgical interventions.[8,11,19–27] And, in rare instances, necessitating a pump exchange.[11,19] The net result of these infectious problems is reduced survival and increased cost, negating the intended benefits of VAD therapy.

Bonde and colleagues[28] examined 286 patients undergoing VAD implants at University of Pittsburgh Medical Center to focus on the incidence and temporal distribution of ESIs (**Table 1**). Actuarial freedom from ESIs at 6 months and 1 year was 60% and 45%, respectively. Between 0 and 3 months, 9.22 ESIs occurred per 100 patient months; at 3 to 6 months, 8.18 ESIs occurred per 100 patient months; and at 6 to 12 months the incidence decreased to 5.38 ESIs per 100 patient months (**Fig. 1**).

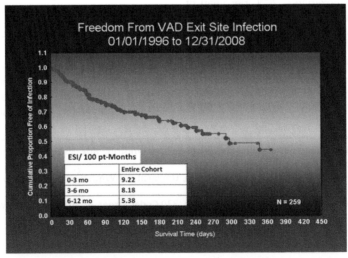

Fig. 1. Freedom from ESI in the entire cohort.

Time to first ESI was predominant in the first 90 days (**Fig. 2**). Recurrent ESIs were twice as common in pulsatile pumps than in continuous-flow VADs. Patients who developed early ESIs proceeded to develop late ESIs (n = 7, 100%).

National Trends in Readmissions After VAD Therapy

Bonde and colleagues[29] examined all adult patients undergoing a primary VAD implant from June 2006 to March 2010 from the prospective data entered in the interagency registry for mechanically assisted circulatory support registry. Patients were excluded who had subsequent right VAD implants or biventricular assist devices. The study examined 1586 patients (355 with a pulsatile pump and 1231 a rotary pump), and involved 192 deaths, 664 patients who were bridged to heart transplant, and 15 who experienced cardiac recovery. By 6 months 55% of patients were free of readmission, with stabilization between 1 and 3 years of 39% to 31% freedom from readmission. Freedom from readmission was not influenced by age, prior neurologic event, diabetes, intention to treat, diagnosis, or INTERMACS profile. Patients with rotary pumps showed significantly higher freedom from readmission beyond 1 year compared with those with pulsatile pumps (45% vs 27%, respectively; $P<.01$). Freedom from readmission was lower for those with ESIs ($P<.01$). The main known causes for first readmission remained ESIs (>70%). Patients who developed ESIs spent more time in the hospital and had 10 times as many readmissions compared with the cohort with no ESIs. Those with ESIs had reduced survival.

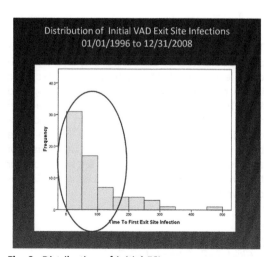

Fig. 2. Distribution of initial ESI.

THE SOLUTION

The solution to the problem is to power the VAD device remotely, thus eliminating the need for a percutaneous driveline. One of the primary aims of National Institutes of Health–funded research to support the development of VAD technology and artificial hearts has been to produce a totally implantable system capable of powering itself remotely with no drivelines traversing the skin. Industry and researchers addressed this using an induction-based transcutaneous energy transfer system (TETS).

Current Limitations of TETS

To address the problem of repeated driveline infections and reduced quality of life from permanently being tethered to a power console, industry and researchers attempted to develop a TETS using induction transfer.[6] However, after several decades of laboratory testing and prototype development, clinical application has been possible in only two systems ([Arrow LionHeart, Reading, PA, USA] and AbioCor TAH [ABIOMED, Inc, Danvers, MA, USA]). Clinical and laboratory experiences have shown several drawbacks with the current TETS technology, namely problems with alignment and the need for the transmitting and receiving coils to be located nearby.[6,7] The system incurs significant energy loss beyond 10 mm separation, resulting in significant heat generation.[7] The need for proximity means that the system must be implanted just under the skin and the external coil must be secured in position with adhesives; this poses various problems associated with skin irritability and thermal injury, which can result in burns. Any of these issues can result in a break in contact and catastrophic energy loss (this was one reason the Arrow LionHeart was withdrawn from the European market, a device which used TETS).[16] Continuous skin contact maintained with adhesives is not practical or clinically feasible, as was learned from transcutaneous drug delivery platforms that require users to change the site of application on a daily basis to prevent skin irritation and subsequent epithelial breakage. Although fraught with problems, the LionHeart trial showed overall reduced infections.

Innovation Through the Free-Range Resonant Electrical Energy Delivery System

Advances in wireless data communication have significantly improved the portability of electronic devices. More recently, wireless power technology offers the possibility of eliminating the remaining wired connection: the power cord. When used with a VAD, wireless power technology will elimi-nate complications and infections caused by the percutaneous wired connection for implanted devices.

Several techniques exist to transmit power wire-lessly from a transmitter to a receiver. For all methods, a tradeoff exists between the amount of power transferred and the separation distance between transmitter and receiver. Microwatts of power can be transferred over kilometer distances at high efficiencies using far-field techniques, whereas hundreds of watts can be transferred over meter distances at high efficiencies using near-field techniques. Some of the existing near-field applications, such as electronic toothbrushes and wireless charging pads, use inductive coupling tech-niques to charge devices over a few centimeters.

The Free-Range Resonant Electrical Energy Delivery (FREE-D) wireless power system uses magnetically coupled resonators to efficiently transfer power across meter distances to a VAD implanted in the human body. The transmit and receive resonators are essentially coils of wire that are tuned to resonate at a specific frequency. The resonator size and shape can be modified to accommodate application specifications, such as room size and patient body geometry. Addition-ally, an adaptive frequency tracking method can be implemented to achieve maximum power transfer efficiency, upwards of 70%, for nearly any angular orientation over a range of separation distances.

AIM

The authors propose to power a VAD device through strong resonant coupling technology, which affords seamless energy supply without compromising mobility or requiring direct contact between the individual and energy source.

SYSTEM OVERVIEW
Circuit Model

Fig. 3 shows a diagram of the basic magnetically coupled resonator wireless power system. The two-element transmitter consists of a single-turn drive resonator and a multiturn resonator that wire-lessly transmits power to a two-element receiver that also consists of a single-turn drive resonator and multiturn resonator, but not necessarily with the same dimensions as the transmitter. These two resonant systems efficiently exchange energy

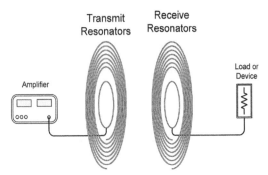

Fig. 3. Schematic of magnetically coupled resonators configuration.

through sharing nonradiative magnetic fields that oscillate at a specific frequency (approximately 7.65 MHz for this VAD application). The most significant interaction occurs between the two multiturn resonators, which are high-Q LCR tank resonators. These resonators share a mutual inductance that is a function of resonator geom-etry and separation distance between the resona-tors. When the receive resonator is within range of the magnetic field generated by the transmitter, power will be transferred wirelessly between the resonators.

Fig. 4 shows the circuit schematic for this system in terms of the lumped circuit elements L, C, and R. The transmit drive resonator and trans-mit multiturn resonator are modeled as inductors L_1 and L_2, and the receive drive resonator and mul-titurn resonator are modeled as inductors L_3 and L_4 respectively. Capacitors C_1 through C_4 are selected so that each magnetically coupled reso-nator will operate at the same resonant frequency according to the following equation:

$$f_{res} = \frac{1}{2\pi\sqrt{L_i C_i}}$$

The resistors R_1 through R_4 represent the para-sitic resistances of the resonators, and are typi-cally less than 1 Ω. Each resonant circuit is linked by the coupling coefficients k_{12}, k_{23}, and k_{34}. These coupling coefficients are typically an order of magnitude greater than the cross-coupling terms (k_{13}, k_{14}, and k_{24}), which have been neglected in the circuit analysis for simplicity. The transfer function shown below for the circuit model in **Fig. 2** is derived using Kirchh-off's voltage law:

$$\frac{V_L}{V_s} = \frac{j\omega^3 k_{12} k_{23} k_{34} L_2 L_3 \sqrt{L_1 L_4 R_L}}{k_{12}^2 k_{34}^2 L_1 L_2 L_3 L_4 \omega^4 + Z_1 Z_2 Z_3 Z_4 + \omega^2 \left(k_{12}^2 L_1 L_2 Z_3 Z_4 + k_{23}^2 L_2 L_3 Z_1 Z_4 + k_{34}^2 L_3 L_4 Z_1 Z_2\right)}$$

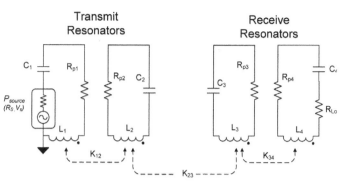

Fig. 4. Equivalent circuit model of the FREE-D system.

$$Z_1 = R_1 + R_3 + j\omega L_1 + \frac{1}{j\omega C_1}$$

$$Z_2 = R_2 + j\omega L_2 + \frac{1}{j\omega C_2}$$

$$Z_3 = R_3 + j\omega L_3 + \frac{1}{j\omega C_3}$$

$$Z_4 = R_4 + R_L + j\omega L_1 + \frac{1}{j\omega C_4}$$

Fig. 5 shows the v-shaped efficiency plateau for the large copper resonators used throughout the experiments discussed later. As the distance between the transmit and receive resonators increases, the amount of coupling between the resonators decreases, and the frequency separation also decreases until the two resonant peaks converge at f_{res}. In the overcoupled regime (distances <0.6 m in **Fig. 5**), the resonators share substantial magnetic flux and the system is capable

of achieving maximum efficiency; in the undercoupled regime (distances >0.6 m in **Fig. 3**), the shared flux decreases below a threshold so that maximum efficiency cannot be achieved. Critical coupling is the point of transition between these two regimes, and corresponds to the greatest range at which maximum efficiency can be achieved. At any distance in the overcoupled regime, two different resonant frequencies are present in the magnetically coupled system, caused by the in-phase and out-of-phase modes of the overlapping magnetic fields. In this region, the efficiency can be maximized through tuning the frequency to the higher of these resonant peaks, as can be seen in the v-shaped curve in **Fig. 3**. In the undercoupled regime, wireless power transfer can still occur, but the maximum achievable efficiency is limited and declines rapidly with distance.

FREE-D System for a VAD

One way to increase the range at which high power transfer efficiency can be achieved is to increase the size of the transmit and receive resonators. However, for use with a VAD, the size of the receive resonator is limited because it will be implanted in the human body. Therefore, another technique using a third relay resonator (**Fig. 6**) is implemented to accommodate greater separation distances between transmit and receive resonators. This relay resonator configuration is a practical design because several transmit resonators could be installed throughout a room (eg, walls, beds, couches, chairs), whereas a single relay resonator could be built into a jacket, much like the HeartMate GoGear Holster Vest (Thoratec Corporation, Pleasanton, California), worn by the patient, which would always be within range of the smaller receive resonator implanted in the patient's body. **Fig. 6** also shows a complete block diagram of the additional circuitry required to use the FREE-D system with a VAD. A radio

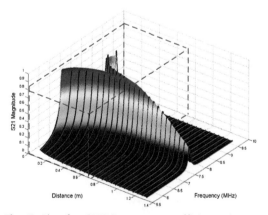

Fig. 5. Plot for FREE-D resonator efficiency (power gain) as a function of resonator separation distance and frequency.

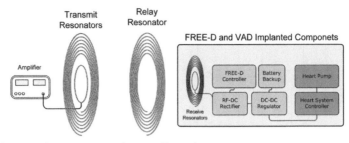

Fig. 6. Schematic of FREE-D for a VAD complete configuration.

frequency–direct current (RF-DC) rectifier is added to the receiver circuit to convert the oscillating RF signal to DC power. A DC-DC regulator steps down this DC voltage to a new DC voltage compatible with the VAD controller and VAD. A backup battery can provide power to the VAD controller intermittently in case FREE-D temporarily delivers insufficient power to the VAD controller. Ideally this battery will be rechargeable so that it can be charged by the FREE-D system with minimal access to the battery itself. This receiver circuitry and experimental configuration is shown in **Figs. 7** and **8**.

SAFETY OF FREE-D SYSTEM

Like all wireless devices, wireless power systems must respect two sets of regulations: electromagnetic interference (EMI) and safety. If the system uses an industrial, scientific, and medical (ISM) frequency band, such as 13.56 MHz, and does not encode data in the power carrier, then it is subject to Federal Communications Commission (FCC) part 18 regulations, and not to FCC part 15 regulations; operating in this fashion, the part 18 EMI regulations do not limit the transmitted power. (Part 18 does place limits on out-of-band emissions; this will require the use of high-quality

waveforms with very little out-of-band energy but, again, does not restrict the power that can be transmitted inside the ISM band.)

The system must of course still respect safety limits. For near-field systems such as FREE-D, compliance with safety regulations must be evaluated in terms of specific absorption rate (SAR), measured in W/kg, and the associated basic restrictions. The use of incident field strength (measured in V/m [electric field] or A/m [magnetic field]) and the associated reference levels significantly overestimate human exposure. In a prior study, the authors collaborated with Dr Niels Kuster of The Foundation for Research on Information Technologies in Society and Eidgenössische Technische Hochschule: The Swiss Federal Institute of Technology, Zurich to numerically calculate SAR in humans for several representative wireless power transmitter configurations. **Fig. 9** shows three representative transmit resonator configurations studied; **Fig. 10** shows calculated SAR. SAR was calculated for four detailed anatomic human models, known as the "virtual family." For the resonator and body geometries studied, 45 W was the lowest transmit power level at which a basic restriction was reached, which is higher than the power level the authors are proposing to use.

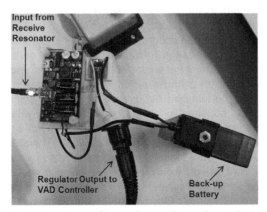

Fig. 7. RF-DC rectifier and DC-DC regulator circuit with back-up battery.

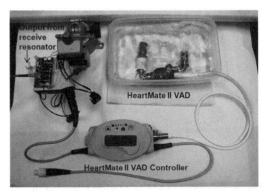

Fig. 8. RF-DC rectifier and DC-DC converter circuit in line with HeartMate II VAD and VAD controller.

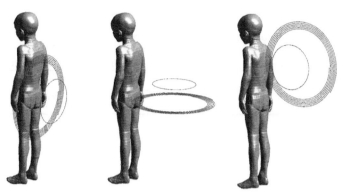

Fig. 9. Three representative resonator configurations studied: coronal, axial, sagittal.

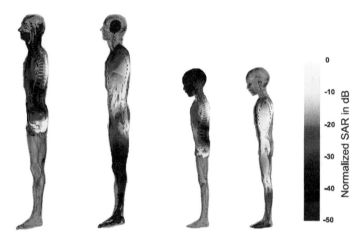

Fig. 10. Local SAR in the models Duke and Thelonius in two sagittal planes (centered and 75 mm off-center) for coronal exposure.

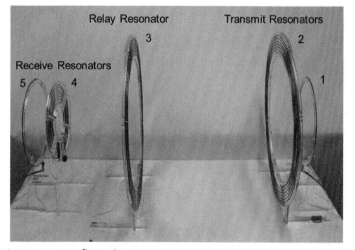

Fig. 11. Experiment 1 resonator configuration.

Table 2 Experiment 1 resonator dimensions and separation distances					
	Resonator 1	Resonator 2	Resonator 3	Resonator 4	Resonator 5
Outer diameter (cm)	31.0	59.0	59.0	28.0	31.0
Distance from 1 (cm)	0.00	6.35	59.7	90.2	100

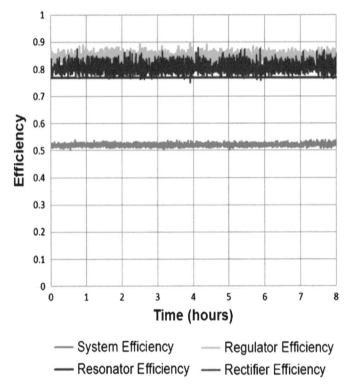

— System Efficiency   — Regulator Efficiency
— Resonator Efficiency   — Rectifier Efficiency

Fig. 12. Experiment 1 efficiency characteristic.

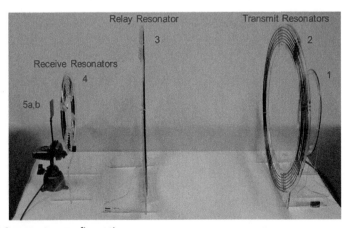

Fig. 13. Experiment 2 resonator configuration.

Table 3
Experiment 2 resonator dimensions and separation distances

	Resonator 1	Resonator 2	Resonator 3	Resonator 4	Resonator 5a	Resonator 5b
Outer diameter (cm)	31.0	59.0	59.0	28.0	5.70	4.30
Distance from 1 (cm)	0.00	6.35	59.7	90.2	99.8	100

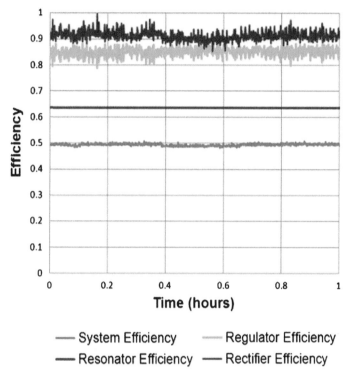

Fig. 14. Experiment 2 efficiency characteristic.

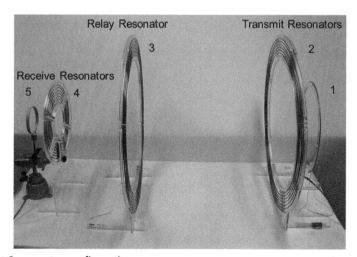

Fig. 15. Experiment 3 resonator configuration.

Table 4
Experiment 3 resonator dimensions and separation distances

	Resonator 1	Resonator 2	Resonator 3	Resonator 4	Resonator 5
Outer diameter (cm)	31.0	59.0	59.0	28.0	9.50
Distance from 1 (cm)	0.00	6.35	59.7	90.2	100

FREE-D EXPERIMENTAL ANALYSIS

The system in **Fig. 6** was experimentally tested using the FREE-D wireless power system and the HeartMate II (Thoratec Corporation) and VentrAssist VADs (VentraCor, Ltd, Chatswood, Australia). Six separate experiments were conducted to monitor the following FREE-D system properties:

1. Power delivery with a static, 1-m separation distance between transmit and receive resonators using both the HeartMate II and VentrAssist VADs.
2. Power delivery throughout an extended duration of FREE-D operation.
3. Temperature of the receive resonator.
4. Power delivery via relay resonators for various receive resonator sizes.

5. Power delivery with a static FREE-D configuration for all VentrAssist VAD pump speeds.

Experiment 1

The configuration for experiment 1 (**Fig. 11**) operated continuously for 8 hours without any loss of power delivered to the left ventricular assist device. The resonator sizes and distances between each resonator can be seen in **Table 2**. The large, copper receive resonator temperature started at 71°F, rose steadily over the course of approximately 1 hour to 82°F, and remained constant for the next 7 hours. The efficiencies (power out divided by power in) for the transmit-receive resonators, RF-DC rectifier, DC-DC regulator, and system efficiency are shown in **Fig. 12**. The data for these efficiency

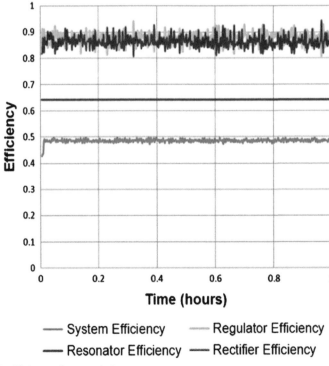

Fig. 16. Experiment 3 efficiency characteristic.

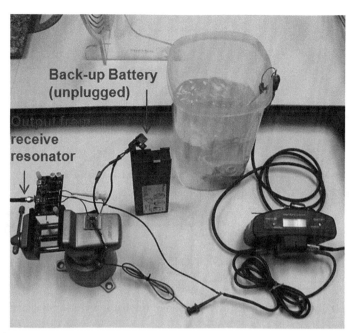

Fig. 17. RF-DC rectifier and DC-DC converter circuit in line with MagLev VAD and VAD (Ventracor, Chatswood, Australia) controller.

Table 5
Experiment 6 resonator dimensions and separation distances

	Resonator 1	Resonator 2	Resonator 3	Resonator 4	Resonator 5
Outer diameter (cm)	31.0	59.0	59.0	28.0	9.50
Distance from 1 (cm)	0.00	12.5	60.7	83.6	90.0

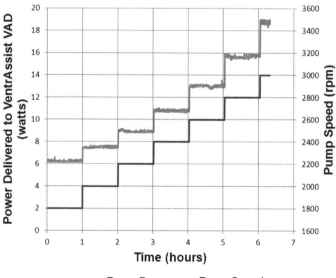

Fig. 18. Pump power and pump speed over 7 hours continuous functioning of a Ventrassist pump, with an uninterrupted power supply by the FREE-D system.

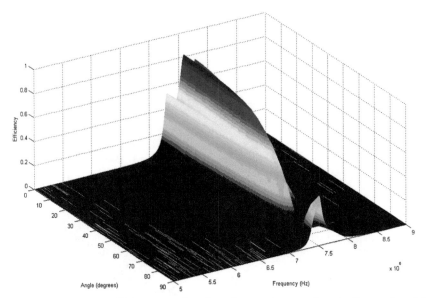

Fig. 19. Plot for FREE-D resonator efficiency as a function of resonator angular misalignment and frequency.

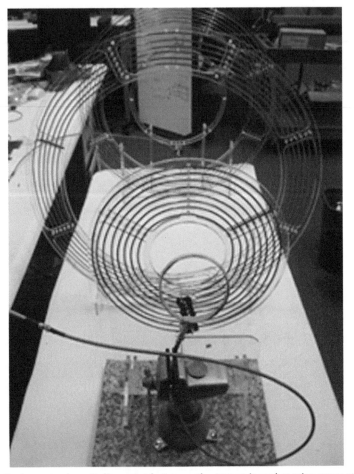

Fig. 20. The effects that an angular misalignment between the transmit and receive resonators have on system efficiency (receive coil facing the transmitting coil).

calculations were logged continuously over the entire 8-hour duration, and the constant efficiency curves verify the successful operation of this experiment.

Experiment 2

The configuration for experiment 2 (**Fig. 13**) operated continuously for 1 hour while using a small, printed circuit board (PCB) receive resonator. The resonator sizes and distances between each resonator can be seen in **Table 3**. The receive PCB resonator temperature rapidly rose to 153°F in 7 minutes, and then remained steady at 146°F for the duration of the experiment. This temperature rise is caused by the properties of the PCB material, and is addressed in experiment 3 using a non-PCB resonator. **Fig. 14** shows the efficiencies for each component in the FREE-D system for this experiment.

Experiment 3

The configuration for experiment 3 (**Fig. 15**) operated continuously for 1 hour. The resonator sizes and distances between each resonator can be seen in **Table 4**. The small, copper receive resonator temperature rose from an initial temperature of 77°F to 87°F in 7 minutes, and then remained constant at 86°F for the duration of the experiment. **Fig. 16** shows the efficiencies for each component in the FREE-D system.

For each experiment, the average rectifier and regulator efficiencies remain nearly the same. Therefore, the system efficiency is primarily controlled by the transmit–receive resonator efficiency, which changes according to the size of the receive resonators used in each experiment. With the large receive resonator in experiment 1, the resonator efficiency is highest, whereas the small PCB resonator has the worst efficiency. Therefore, the smaller the receive resonator, the more sensitive the power efficiency will be to misalignments between the relay resonator

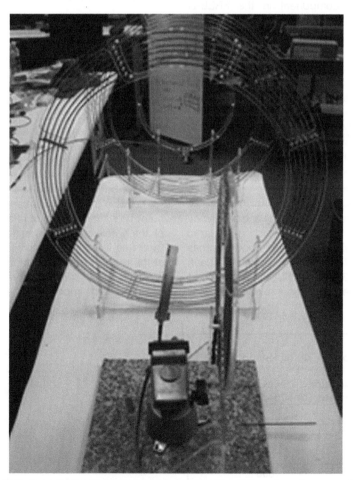

Fig. 21. The effects that an angular misalignment between the transmit and receive resonators have on system efficiency (receive coil at right angles to the transmitting coil).

embedded in a vest and the receive resonator implanted in the body.

Experiment 4

The configuration for experiment 4 (**Fig. 17**) operated continuously for 2 weeks over a full range of pump speeds for the VentrAssist Magnetic Levitation VAD (Ventracor, Ltd). The resonators used were identical to those in experiment 3 (see **Fig. 15**); however, the separation distances were modified slightly, as can be seen in **Table 5**. These modified separation distances allow for a resonator efficiency of 90% or greater. Data were logged using the VentrAssist VentraView VV10_0 software. Also, the VAD pump speed was varied from 1800 to 3000 revolutions per minute (rpm) by increments of 200 rpm. As the pump speed increases, the power demanded by the pump also increases. Therefore, the input power to the transmit resonator was increased manually each time the pump speed was increased to meet the power needs of the VAD. **Fig. 18** shows the efficiencies for each component in the FREE-D system over the full 2-week duration of the experiment for the varying pump speeds.

Experiment 5

The configuration for experiment 5 (same as experiment 3 as shown in **Fig. 15**) shows the effects that an angular misalignment between the transmit and receive resonators have on system efficiency. **Fig. 19** shows the relationship between efficiency and angular misalignment, and **Figs. 20** and **21** show the experimental configuration.

Experiment 6

Experiment 6 shows how efficiency and frequency tuning are affected when ham (which is similar in electrical conductivity to the human body) comes in close proximity to the receive resonator. Each slab of ham is 17.33-mm thick, with an approximated capacitance of C_{HAM} = picofarads Two

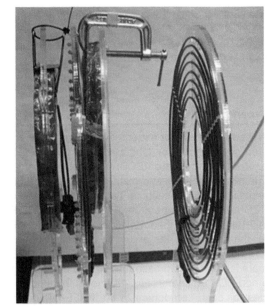

Fig. 22. Insulated copper resonators with ham in physical contact with the receive resonator.

different materials and sizes of resonators were tested in this experiment, as outlined in **Table 6** and shown in **Figs. 22** and **23**.

Several different configurations were tested to determine whether the presence of ham will have a negative effect on resonator efficiency: no ham present, ham nearby resonators, ham in physical contact with the resonators, and metal nearby the resonators. **Figs. 24** and **25** compare the effects on efficiency for each of these configurations for both resonators tested.

The ham's ability to detune the receive resonator has a more harmful effect on the efficiency of the wireless power transfer than its potential to act as a flux interceptor. However, regardless of the reason, the quality factor of the resonators is reduced for all configurations. Coil design becomes very important when considering how

Table 6
Experiment 6 resonator characteristics

	Resonator Diameter (cm)	Resonator Capacitance (pF)
Insulated (blue) copper resonators	28.0	25.0
PCB resonators	4.30	1000

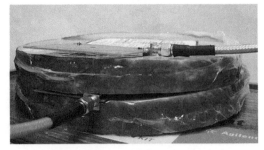

Fig. 23. PCB resonators with ham in physical contact with the receive resonator.

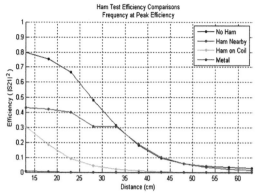

Fig. 24. Experiment 6 efficiency insulated (*blue*) copper resonator efficiency analysis.

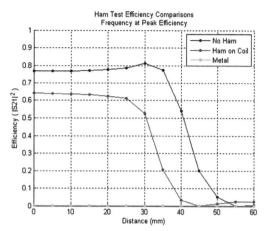

Fig. 25. Experiment 6 efficiency PCB resonator efficiency analysis.

to minimize the detuning effect when ham or human body tissue comes within close range of the receive resonator. Increasing the inductance of a resonator is desirable to maximize the quality factor Q of a coil. However, if the inductance is so large that the required trimming capacitance of the resonator for the desired resonant frequency $\left(f = 1/2\pi\sqrt{LC} \right)$ is on the same order of magnitude as the capacitance of the ham, the efficiency of the system will be worse. Research must be performed on the capacitance of the tissues in the human body where the resonators are likely to be implanted to determine a minimum threshold for trimming capacitance and an ideal balance between *L* and *C* of the resonators when considering optimal resonator designs. Impedance matching techniques may solve the

reduced efficiency with ham present for the PCB resonators.

SUMMARY

The authors' vision constitutes a completely implantable cardiac assist system affording tether-free mobility in an unrestricted space powered wirelessly by the innovative FREE-D system (**Fig. 26**). Patients will have no power drivelines traversing the skin, and this system will allow power to be delivered over room distances and will eliminate trouble-prone wirings, bulky consoles, and replaceable batteries.

The authors envisage converting living spaces to a safe all-encompassing environment in which patients are able to receive power no matter whether they are in their home, office, or car. This system is

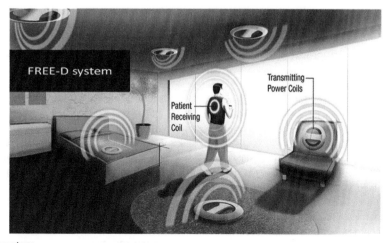

Fig. 26. FREE-D system.

unlike any older TET system, which had the disadvantages of reliability, contact burns, or irritation. The advantages of the FREE-D system range from reduced potential for life-threatening infections, better patient safety, and improved quality of life.

REFERENCES

1. Deng MC, Edwards LB, Hertz MI, et al. Mechanical circulatory support device database of the International Society for Heart and Lung Transplantation: first annual report–2003. J Heart Lung Transplant 2003;22(6):653–62.
2. Holman WL, Kormos RL, Naftel DC, et al. Predictors of death and transplant in patients with a mechanical circulatory support device: a multi-institutional study. J Heart Lung Transplant 2009;28(1):44–50.
3. Miller LW, Pagani FD, Russell SD, et al. HeartMate II Clinical Investigators. Use of a continuous-flow device in patients awaiting heart transplantation. N Engl J Med 2007;357(9):885–96.
4. Pagani FD, Miller LW, Russell SD, et al. HeartMate II Investigators. Extended mechanical circulatory support with a continuous-flow rotary left ventricular assist device. J Am Coll Cardiol 2009;54(4):312–21.
5. Slaughter MS, Rogers JG, Milano CA, et al. HeartMate II Investigators. Advanced heart failure treated with continuous-flow left ventricular assist device. N Engl J Med 2009;361(23):2241–51.
6. Genovese EA, Dew MA, Teuteberg JJ, et al. Incidence and patterns of adverse event onset during the first 60 days after ventricular assist device implantation. Ann Thorac Surg 2009; 88(4):1162–70.
7. Martin SI, Wellington L, Stevenson KB, et al. Effect of body mass index and device type on infection in left ventricular assist device support beyond 30 days. Interact Cardiovasc Thorac Surg 2010;11(1): 20–3.
8. Holman WL, Pamboukian SV, McGiffin DC, et al. Device related infections: are we making progress? J Card Surg 2010;25(4):478–83.
9. Raymond AL, Kfoury AG, Bishop CJ, et al. Obesity and left ventricular assist device driveline exit site infection. ASAIO J 2010;56(1):57–60.
10. Zierer A, Melby SJ, Voeller RK, et al. Late-onset driveline infections: the Achilles' heel of prolonged left ventricular assist device support. Ann Thorac Surg 2007;84(2):515–20.
11. Allen JG, Weiss ES, Schaffer JM, et al. Quality of life and functional status in patients surviving 12 months after left ventricular assist device implantation. J Heart Lung Transplant 2010;29(3):278–85.
12. Wilson W, Taubert KA, Gewitz M, et al. Prevention of infective endocarditis. J Am Dent Assoc 2008; 139(Suppl):3S–24S.
13. Baddour LM, Bettmann MA, Bolger AF, et al. Nonvalvular cardiovascular device-related infections. Circulation 2003;108(16):2015–31.
14. Kurtz SM, Lau E, Schmier J, et al. Infection burden for hip and knee arthroplasty in the United States. J Arthroplasty 2008;23(7):984–91.
15. Holman WL, Park SJ, Long JW, et al. REMATCH Investigators. Infection in permanent circulatory support: experience from the REMATCH trial. J Heart Lung Transplant 2004;23(12):1359–65.
16. Gordon RJ, Quagliarello B, Lowy FD. Ventricular assist device-related infections. Lancet Infect Dis 2006;6(7):426–37.
17. Monkowski DH, Axelrod P, Fekete T, et al. Infections associated with ventricular assist devices: epidemiology and effect on prognosis after transplantation. Transpl Infect Dis 2007;9(2):114–20.
18. Baddour LM, Epstein AE, Erickson CC, et al. Update on cardiovascular implantable electronic device infections and their management: a scientific statement from the American Heart Association. Circulation 2010;121(3):458–77.
19. Schaffer JM, Allen JG, Weiss ES, et al. Infectious complications after pulsatile-flow and continuous-flow left ventricular assist device implantation. J Heart Lung Transplant 2011;30(2):164–74.
20. Topkara VK, Kondareddy S, Malik F, et al. Infectious complications in patients with left ventricular assist device: etiology and outcomes in the continuous-flow era. Ann Thorac Surg 2010;90(4):1270–7.
21. Siegenthaler MP, Martin J, Pernice K, et al. The Jarvik 2000 is associated with less infections than the HeartMate left ventricular assist device. Eur J Cardiothorac Surg 2003;23(5):748–54 [discussion: 754–5].
22. Holman WL, Kirklin JK, Naftel DC, et al. Infection after implantation of pulsatile mechanical circulatory support devices. J Thorac Cardiovasc Surg 2010; 139(6):1632, e2–6.
23. Dew MA, Kormos RL, Winowich S, et al. Human factors issues in ventricular assist device recipients and their family caregivers. ASAIO J 2000;46(3): 367–73.
24. Kormos RL, Teuteberg JJ, Pagani FD, et al. HeartMate II Clinical Investigators. Right ventricular failure in patients with the HeartMate II continuous-flow left ventricular assist device: incidence, risk factors, and effect on outcomes. J Thorac Cardiovasc Surg 2010;139(5):1316–24.
25. Hravnak M, George E, Kormos RL. Management of chronic left ventricular assist device percutaneous lead insertion sites. J Heart Lung Transplant 1993; 12(5):856–63.
26. Haj-Yahia S, Birks EJ, Rogers P, et al. Midterm experience with the Jarvik 2000 axial flow left ventricular assist device. J Thorac Cardiovasc Surg 2007; 134(1):199–203.

27. El-Banayosy A, Arusoglu L, Kizner L, et al. Preliminary experience with the LionHeart left ventricular assist device in patients with end-stage heart failure. Ann Thorac Surg 2003;75(5):1469–75.

28. Bonde P, Bermudez C, Lockard KL, et al. The Ventricular Assist Device (VAD) Driveline: What is The Price of Living with This Technology? International Society of Heart Lung Transplantation. 30th Annual Meeting and Scientific Sessions. Chicago, 2010.

29. Bonde P, Dew MA, Meyer D, et al. National Trends in Readmission (REA) Rates Following Left Ventricular Assist Device (LVAD) Therapy, International Society of Heart Lung Transplantation. 31st Annual Meeting. San Diego, April 15, 2011.

Editorial Comments on "Towards Total Implantability Using FREE-D System: Achieving Un-Tethered VAD Operation Over Large Distances"

John A. Elefteriades, MD

KEY CONCEPTS

Dr Pramod Bonde and colleagues clearly state the shortcomings of an external driveline from the ventricular assist device (VAD) to the exterior. The investigators elegantly state the case for untethering. Many of us feel that infection is inevitable as long as the integument is pierced; so, we strongly support the crusade to achieve "wireless" transmission of energy. It is important to realize that we are not talking about transmission of information, but, rather, the transmission of substantive amounts of energy. It is valuable to keep in mind that our group at Yale has used radiofrequency radio transmission of energy across the intact skin for more than 4 decades, since the inception of the technique by Glenn and Hogan.[1,2] We use this for powering our diaphragm pacemakers (**Fig. 1**). We are not simply telemetering data but providing all the energy for pulse train stimulation of the diaphragm. So, there is a long track record of feasibility in humans, without skin damage or loss of the life-sustaining stimuli.

STRENGTHS

The case for achieving relief from tethering is compelling. The engineering is exciting. This work will ultimately represent a giant leap forward in VAD technology, a step we believe will be even bigger than miniaturization and rotary pumping.

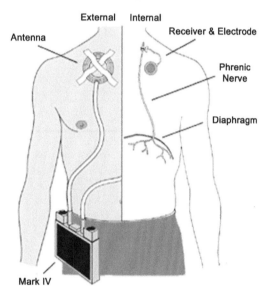

Fig. 1. Diaphragm pacing system. (*Courtesy of* Avery, Long Island, NY, USA; with permission.)

Section of Cardiac Surgery, Yale University School of Medicine, Boardman 2, 333 Cedar Street, New Haven, CT 06510, USA
E-mail address: john.elefteriades@yale.edu

Cardiol Clin 29 (2011) 627–628
doi:10.1016/j.ccl.2011.07.007
0733-8651/11/$ – see front matter © 2011 Published by Elsevier Inc.

WEAKNESSES

As is clear from the "ham steak" experiments, which thwarted the transmission of energy, this technology is not yet ready for prime time.

REFERENCES

1. Glenn WW, Phelps ML, Elefteriades JA, et al. Twenty years of experience in phrenic nerve stimulation to pace the diaphragm. Pacing Clin Electrophysiol 1986;9(6 Pt 1):780–4.
2. Elefteriades JA, Quin JA, Hogan JF, et al. Long-term follow-up of pacing of the conditioned diaphragm in quadriplegia. Pacing Clin Electrophysiol 2002;25(6): 897–906.

Right Ventricular Dysfunction in Patients Undergoing Left Ventricular Assist Device Implantation: Predictors, Management, and Device Utilization

Abeel A. Mangi, MD*

KEYWORDS

- Right ventricular dysfunction
- Nonreversible right ventricular failure
- Left ventricular support device • Biventricular support

Right ventricular dysfunction occurs fairly frequently during the conduct of standard cardiac operations, but is largely a reversible and transient phenomenon. It is generally thought to be caused by embolization of air down the right coronary artery, incomplete or inadequate revascularization, or inadequate myocardial protection. Conventional and widely used strategies such as reperfusing the heart at higher blood pressure, revascularization, or "resting" the empty beating heart on bypass are known to ameliorate the severity of this condition.

For the purposes of this article, the authors define nonreversible failure of the right ventricle as the need for postoperative inotropic support for greater than 14 days, inhaled nitric oxide for greater than 48 hours, right-sided circulatory support, or hospital discharge on an inotrope. Nonreversible failure of the right ventricle represents the more malignant form of this syndrome, and is seen in 0.04% to 0.1% of postcardiotomy cases. Unfortunately, the incidence of right ventricular dysfunction after left ventricular assist device (LVAD) implantation that fails to resolve in the operating room is reported as frequently as 20% to 50% and imposes a considerable burden in terms of postoperative morbidity and mortality. Should this syndrome supervene, the mortality of an LVAD operation increases from 19% to 43%.[1–3] Although most patients can be maintained with prolonged inotropic support, 10% to 15% may require implantation of a separate right ventricular support device (RVAD).

THE IMPLICATIONS OF RIGHT VENTRICULAR DYSFUNCTION

Persistent right ventricular dysfunction after LVAD implantation has been shown to independently predict higher incidences of end-organ dysfunction, longer intensive care unit and hospital lengths of stay, increased morbidity, and increased mortality in patients awaiting transplantation.[2,4,5] Right ventricular dysfunction severe enough to

Division of Cardiac Surgery, Yale University School of Medicine, 330 Cedar Street, BB 204, New Haven, CT 06510, USA
* Division of Cardiac Surgery, Temple University Hospital, Suite 301, Parkinson Pavilion, 3401 North Broad Street, Philadelphia, PA 19040.
E-mail address: abeel.mangi@yale.edu

Cardiol Clin 29 (2011) 629–637
doi:10.1016/j.ccl.2011.08.003
0733-8651/11/$ – see front matter © 2011 Published by Elsevier Inc.

require RVAD implantation is independently predictive of death.

Impaired Hepatic Perfusion

Patients who require LVAD implantation have tenuous end-organ function, usually because of both right and left ventricular failure. It has been well recognized that blood flow is distributed away from splanchnic organs in the setting of systemic hypotension, such as may occur in a patients with severe left-sided heart failure. This diversion of flow is accomplished by mesenteric vasoconstriction, which in turn leads to decrease in portal venous return to the liver. Because the majority of oxygen flow to the liver comes from the portal circulation, this can result in centrilobular necrosis and a resultant release of hepatic enzymes. The need to place such a patient on cardiopulmonary bypass with attendant hypotension and hemodilution exacerbates mesenteric vasoconstriction, furthering liver injury by the mechanisms discussed earlier.[6,7]

When right-sided heart failure occurs in addition to left-sided heart failure, the addition of "passive hepatic congestion," which might more accurately be termed venous hypertension of the liver, serves to exacerbate hepatic hypoxia, because the column of low-pressure portal venous blood cannot negotiate the high-pressure column of venous blood and can no longer perfuse the hepatocytes. The addition of right-sided failure therefore serves to exacerbate hepatic hypoxia already present because of left-sided heart failure. This is one explanation as to why, even after correcting left ventricular performance with cardiac replacement therapies, the overwhelming majority of patients (in some estimates as high as 94%) demonstrate persistent hepatic dysfunction.[8]

Systemic Inflammatory Response Due to Splanchnic Hypoperfusion

More troubling is the systemic inflammatory response that hepatic dysfunction can engender. Rossi and colleagues[9] studied 11 randomly selected patients with normal cardiac chamber size and function who were undergoing elective isolated coronary artery bypass graft surgery with the use of cardiopulmonary bypass. In the absence of significant macrocirculatory changes and postoperative complications, a correlation existed between the damage to the gastrointestinal mucosa, subsequent increased permeability, *Escherichia coli* bacteremia, and the activation of a self-limited inflammatory response. In the liver sinusoid, free intravascular lipopolysaccharide (LPS) produced from degradation of the bacterial

cell wall binds to LPS-binding protein (LBP). This complex has a high affinity for the CD14 cell-surface receptor on the Kupffer cell, causing activation and secretion of inflammatory cytokines including, but not limited to, tumor necrosis factor (TNF)-α, interleukin (IL)-1β, and IL-6; eicosanoids; intercellular adhesion molecules; platelet-activating factor; oxygen free radicals; and nitric oxide. Simultaneously, soluble CD14 binds with the LPS/LBP complex and activates endothelial cells, which then release a similar inflammatory cascade. The secretion of TNF-α sets in motion the cellular, metabolic, and vascular responses of systemic inflammatory response syndromes, septic shock, and multiple-system organ failure syndromes.[10] Although transient splanchnic ischemia may be self-limiting and clinically irrelevant in relatively healthy patients with normal hepatic function, this does not hold true for patients with end-stage heart disease who already have severely compromised liver function. In fact, this has been demonstrated by Masai and colleagues.[11] Studying a group of 16 patients undergoing LVAD implantation, they found that patients with hyperbilirubinemia and inflammatory reactions before LVAD support showed worsening of hyperbilirubinemia, inflammatory cytokine, and hyaluronan levels, despite adequate hemodynamics achieved under LVAD support. These results suggest that inflammatory response contributes to subsequent aggravation of hepatic dysfunction, with cholestasis and fibrosis, and with ongoing derangement in hepatic sinusoidal microcirculation even under adequate systemic circulatory support.[11] Whether such a syndrome can be ameliorated by the use of antibodies to TNF-α, or by empiric use of drugs known to blunt the systemic inflammatory response syndrome, such as Xigris, is speculative and needs to be considered in light of the specific complications that these drugs carry.

Prolonged Hospital Stay and Greater Mortality Awaiting Transplant

Irrespective of what the causes of right-sided failure after LVAD implantation are, it is indisputable that a prolonged requirement for inotropic support translates into a longer intensive care unit stay and a longer overall hospital stay, as well as a greater mortality rate. Kawarana and colleagues[2] have demonstrated that patients who suffer right ventricular dysfunction after LVAD implantation have higher postoperative creatinine (2.2 vs 1.5 mg/dL), greater need for postoperative continuous venovenous hemodialysis (73% vs 26%), greater transfusion requirement (43.2 vs

24.7 units of packed red blood cells), greater requirement for platelet transfusion (58 vs 30 units), longer intensive care unit stay (33 days vs 9 days), and higher mortality (42.8% vs 14.5%).

Of most interest, the higher mortality rate persists even after inotropes have been successfully weaned off, and this mortality is directly correlated with the duration of inotropic support.[4] When Schenk and colleagues[4] examined 176 patients who underwent isolated LVAD implantation, they noted that although 100% of patients were on inotropes on the day of operation, when they could be discontinued, this was most often accomplished between postoperative days 3 and 5. By postoperative day 7, 57% of patients were still inotrope dependent; by postoperative day 14, 33% of patients were still inotrope dependent; and by postoperative day 21, 22% of patients were still inotrope dependent. Patients with nonischemic causes of heart failure, and those with right ventricular stroke work indices less than 500 mm Hg/mL/m^2, were most likely to be on inotropes for longer than 14 days. Most striking, however, was the finding that duration of inotropic support affected 6-month survival. Specifically, patients who tolerated discontinuation of inotropic support on the first postoperative day had a 6-month survival of 72%; but those who required inotropic support until postoperative days 10, 30, and 60 had 6-month survival of 64%, 57%, and 46%, respectively.

Morgan and colleagues[5] suggest that timing of RVAD implantation influences survival to transplantation, likely reflecting a selection bias in candidates for LVAD support and heightened vigilance in the immediate postoperative course. These investigators demonstrated that survival to transplant in patients who underwent early RVAD implantation (ie, within 24 hours) was 70%, versus a survival rate of 57% in those who underwent RVAD implantation greater than 24 hours after LVAD implantation. This finding is statistically significant (P<.001).

In addition, Morgan and colleagues[5] demonstrated that the diminishment in survival when right ventricular support is needed persists after transplantation. Patients who require RVAD in addition to LVAD have a 1-, 5-, and 10-year posttransplant actuarial survival rate of 71.4%, 71.4%, and 71.4%, respectively, whereas patients requiring LVAD only have a posttransplant actuarial survival rate of 90.5%, 80.4%, and 78.5 at 1, 5, and 10 years. While this discussion of right ventricular failure is therefore germane to patients being bridged to transplantation, it is of even more importance in destination therapy patients, in whom transplantation is not an option and in whom appropriate selection is critically important.

Mortality After RVAD Implantation

Right ventricular failure of a magnitude that requires RVAD implantation emerges as an independent predictor of death in every series on the subject. In the series from Frazier and colleagues,[12] 4 of 34 patients undergoing LVAD implantation as bridge to transplant required RVAD placement, and none survived to transplantation. In the analysis, right ventricular failure was the only variable that correlated with a negative outcome. Echoing these results, Goldstein and colleagues[13] reported that 21 of 22 patients requiring RVAD died awaiting transplantation, and Kormos and colleagues[14] reported that 40% of patients requiring right ventricular support succumbed before transplantation. In the Cleveland Clinic series, 16 patients required RVAD implantation within 2 days of LVAD implantation, and the remaining 2 required RVAD implantation on postoperative days 3 and 12 because of respiratory failure followed by severe right ventricular dysfunction. High-dose inotropic support preceded RVAD implantation in 17 of 18 patients. Survival to transplantation decreased dramatically with time in this cohort, and was 47% at postoperative day 10, 29% at postoperative day 20, and only 22% at postoperative day 30. Overall, survival to transplant was 27% versus 83% in patients who did not require RVAD implantation.[4]

PREDICTORS OF RIGHT VENTRICULAR DYSFUNCTION AFTER LVAD IMPLANTATION

Right ventricular dysfunction after LVAD implantation is common, is difficult to control, and may have disastrous clinical and programmatic implications. It is intuitive, therefore, that by identifying patients at risk for right ventricular dysfunction, preoperative maneuvers may be undertaken to reduce the likelihood of postoperative right ventricular dysfunction, and that in patients deemed prohibitive risks, alternative means of biventricular support such as the total artificial heart be considered. Consensus is starting to emerge in the literature on which preoperative symptom complex constitutes a high risk for postoperative right ventricular dysfunction.

In general, two schools of thought dominate the discussion of, and approach to, preoperative risk factors for right ventricular failure after LVAD implantation. The first emphasizes patient characteristics and features and the other emphasizes analysis of hemodynamic parameters. From a - practical perspvective, both factors probably carry equal weight and should be considered while evaluating a patient for mechanical circulatory support.

Clinical Predictors of Right Ventricular Failure

Kormos and colleagues[15] have argued that nonhemodynamic preoperative clinical factors are more predictive of right ventricular failure because "patients who are more clinically compromised and have more marginal end-organ function tend to require more extensive right ventricular support after LVAS implantation." Studying 32 patients, these investigators demonstrated that patients with borderline multiorgan failure, elevation of bilirubin or creatinine, a fever around the time of implantation, a requirement for pure pressors, adult respiratory distress syndrome, or right ventricular infarction are at exceedingly high risk for perioperative right ventricular failure requiring prolonged inotropic support or right-sided circulatory support.

This view has been echoed by Pagani and colleagues[16] who, in a study of 32 patients, suggested that there was a higher tendency to develop right ventricular failure necessitating mechanical assistance after LVAD implant in patients who came to medical attention in cardiac arrest, with severe hemodynamic instability (systolic blood pressure ≤75 mm Hg) requiring short-term circulatory support with extracorporeal membrane oxygenation (ECMO), and with evidence of multiorgan failure (defined as serum creatinine level >3 mg/dL or oliguria; international normalized ratio >1.5, or transaminases >5 times normal, or total bilirubin >3 mg/dL; and needing mechanical ventilation).

Recently Fukamachi and colleagues[17] analyzed 100 patients, Ochiai and colleagues[18] studied 245 patients, and Matthews and colleagues[19] looked at 197 patients undergoing LVAD implantation. Using univariate analyses, all 3 investigators have suggested that patient-specific factors do indeed predict the need for prolonged right ventricular inotropic support and/or RVAD. Common factors identified by all 3 investigators include: small body surface area, female sex (which may be a surrogate for smaller body surface area), younger patient age, the presence of myocarditis, and higher preoperative levels of serum aspartate transaminase (AST) levels (637 vs 146, P = .0059).

Additional factors identified separately by the 3 investigators using univariate analysis include the following. Fukamachi and colleagues[17] identified the need for preoperative use of intra-aortic balloon counterpulsation, ECMO, short-term mechanical support, positive pressure ventilation, body temperature, and renal function as assayed by blood urea nitrogen or creatinine as predictive of the need for right-sided mechanical support. Ochiai and colleagues[18] identified the need for preoperative mechanical ventilation (83% vs 56%, P = .015) and preoperative circulatory assistance (48% vs 18%, P = .003) as predictive of the need for prolonged postoperative inotropic support. Matthews and colleagues[19] identified the presence of renal replacement therapy (odds ratio 9.93), dependence on vasopressin (odds ratio 7.24), serum creatinine greater than 2.3 (odds ratio 5.56), dependence on neosynephrine (odds ratio 3.59), serum bilirubin greater than 2 (odds ratio 3.59), serum AST greater than 80 (odds ratio 3.2), a white blood cell count greater than 12,200 (odds ratio 3.36), dependence on ventilator (odds ratio 3.18), need for preoperative mechanical circulatory support ECMO/Tandem/Abiomed (odds ratio 3.17), prior cerebrovascular event (odds ratio 2.99), cardiopulmonary arrest within 24 hours of operation (odds ratio 2.61), and dependence on intravenous antiarrhythmic therapy (odds ratio 2.56) as predictive of right ventricular failure.[19]

On multivariate analysis, Fukamachi and colleagues[17] and Ochiai and colleagues[18] demonstrated that the need for preoperative circulatory support (odds ratio 5.3), female gender (odds ratio 4.5), and nonischemic etiology of cardiogenic shock (odds ratio 3.3) were strongly predictive of the need for postoperative right-sided circulatory support.

On multivariate analysis, Matthews and colleagues[19] demonstrated that a pressor requirement (weighted to receive 4 points), elevation in creatinine (weighted to receive 3 points), elevation in bilirubin (weighted to receive 2.5 points), and elevation in AST (weighted to receive 2 points) strongly predicted postoperative right ventricular failure. The scoring system developed by Matthews and colleagues[19] predicts that patients with a score greater than 5.5 have a 15-fold greater chance of developing right ventricular failure when compared with patients with a score of less than 3.

Although very sophisticated, for practical purposes the Matthews scale is not very different from the earlier descriptions of preoperative predictions of right ventricular failure after LVAD implantation described earlier in this section—that is, patients in hemodynamic extremis with evidence of hepatic or renal dysfunction are at prohibitively high odds for right ventricular failure after LVAD implantation, and are probably best served with institution of biventricular support at initial operation.

Hemodynamic Predictors of Right Ventricular Failure

Right heart catheterization before LVAD implantation has been used to ascertain what, if any, hemodynamic factors are predictive of right ventricular failure. Ochiai and colleagues[18] demonstrated by univariate analysis that patients requiring RVAD had lower mean pulmonary artery pressure (PAP) (33 vs 37 mm Hg, $P = .04$); lower diastolic PAP (25 vs 29 mm Hg, $P = .03$), and lower right ventricular stroke work (543 vs 780 mm Hg/mL, $P = .037$). These results were verified by Fukamachi and colleagues[17] who, using univariate analyses, demonstrated that lower cardiac output (2.8 vs 3.5 L/min, $P = .019$), lower mean PAP (31 vs 38 mm Hg, $P = .015$), and lower right ventricular stroke work index (RVSWI) (151 vs 368 mm Hg/mL/m^2, $P = .011$) were all predictive of postoperative RVAD support. RVSWI in particular emerged as a highly specific predictor, with a specificity of 100%, sensitivity of 54%, positive predictive value of 100%, and negative predictive value of 20%. This finding is also borne out by Matthews and colleagues[19] who demonstrated that an RVSWI of less than 450 has an odds ratio of 2.32 in predicting postoperative failure of the right ventricle, and that a pulmonary artery systolic pressure greater than 50 is protective against postoperative right ventricular failure, with an odds ratio of 0.49. Similarly, Morgan and colleagues[5] suggest that a high central venous pressure (CVP) coupled with low PAP and a low RVSWI are predictive of right ventricular failure after LVAD implantation. In fact it has been demonstrated that patients without pulmonary hypertension were more likely to develop right ventricular failure and die[20] after LVAD implantation.

Farrar and colleagues[21] reported that only 46% of patients with ischemic cardiomyopathy required RVAD whereas 63% of patients with nonischemic cardiomyopathy required RVAD. Alternatively, 46% of patients with biventricular assist devices had nonischemic etiology as opposed to 40% with ischemic cardiomyopathy. In addition, RVAD patients had a higher incidence of reoperation for bleeding (57% vs 27%, $P = .003$), had poorer survival to transplantation (17% vs 74%, $P<.001$) and required LVAD support for 94 days as opposed to 27 days in the no-RVAD group ($P = .002$). The low PAP and low RVSWI are referred to again, implying that depressed right ventricular contractility before LVAD insertion was not strong enough to elevate PAP in the presence of high pulmonary vascular resistance (PVR).

The implications of these findings are that when right ventricular contractility is inadequate to generate a high PAP, the right ventricle is incapable of coping with the changes imposed by LVAD implantation. However, irreversibility of pulmonary hypertension, particularly when associated with high right atrial pressure, may suggest concomitant pulmonary disease or irreversible injury to the right ventricle. In such cases, a 4- to 8-week long trial of selective pulmonary vasodilators (milrinone, sildenafil, prostaglandins) with serial right heart catheterization may be warranted in an attempt to lower PVR and improve cardiac index.

In summary, therefore, patients with nonischemic cardiomyopathy, with a hemodynamic profile suggesting elevation in CVP, diminution of PAP, and a low RVSWI, and with a clinical profile that suggests the need for vasopressors, mechanical support, renal, respiratory, or hepatic dysfunction are at extremely high risk for post-LVAD right-sided heart failure, and should be considered for a priori biventricular support.

Assessment of Right Ventricular Geometry, Function, and Tricuspid Valve Regurgitation

Preimplant echocardiographic assessment of the right ventricle offers an important guide to preoperative and intraoperative management of right ventricular function. A dilated right ventricle that has lost its triangular "wedge-shaped" configuration on a zero-degree 4-chamber view and assumes a globular shape is of concern. It is important to assess the contribution by the basal, free wall, and apical segments of the right ventricle, as well as the position of the interatrial septum and interventricular septum when actuating a continuous-flow LVAD. Excessive unloading of the left ventricle causes the interventricular septum to shift leftward, which in turn induces a series of disadvantageous geometric changes in the right ventricle that eliminate the septal contribution to right ventricular stroke volume. In addition, the annulus of the tricuspid valve that corresponds to the septal leaflet is distorted, perhaps resulting in worsening tricuspid regurgitation.

The presence of severe functional tricuspid regurgitation is often an indicator of severe right ventricular dysfunction that is due to long-standing volume and pressure overload. Therefore, a reluctance to repair the tricuspid valve often exists, owing to concern over exacerbating right ventricular dysfunction. However, clinicians are now realizing that severe preoperative tricuspid insufficiency is a risk factor for early right ventricular failure. The mechanism behind this may be acute and overwhelming volume and pressure overload of the right ventricle. Because of the low pressure sink in the systemic venous chambers, blood would preferentially stream into the systemic venous chambers instead of into the pressurized pulmonary circuit. Accordingly, left-sided chambers (and therefore the LVAD) would remain underfilled, which would potentiate the inability of the device to unload the pulmonary circuit, resulting in a tight spiral of early and overwhelming right ventricular failure. Accordingly, severe tricuspid regurgitation should be repaired or treated with rigid annuloplasty. Destruction of tricuspid leaflets may require valvular replacement, but this is unusual.

Mild to moderate tricuspid regurgitation and a functional valve would probably improve with a reduction in right ventricular afterload that typically occurs during LVAD support.

If the right ventricle is ischemic, consideration should be given to surgical revascularization at the time of LVAD implantation.

PATHOPHYSIOLOGY OF RIGHT VENTRICULAR DYSFUNCTION

There are 4 fundamental causes by which the right ventricle fails after implantation of an LVAD: ischemia, alterations in interventricular balance, position of the interventricular septum, and the need to simultaneously perform volume and pressure work.

Ischemia of the right ventricle or the interventricular septum can occur in a patient with unrevascularized ischemic cardiomyopathy, or when the intracavitary pressure of a distended and overloaded right ventricle exceeds coronary perfusion pressure. Ways in which this situation can be avoided are by revascularizing the right coronary artery at the time of LVAD implantation, or by separating from bypass with a volume underloaded right ventricle, and at a high systemic blood pressure.

In general, under conditions that assume a balanced circulation, left ventricular output must by necessity be equal to right ventricular output. When an LVAD is implanted, it introduces an imbalance in interventricular balance such that the right ventricle must now match LVAD output. In patients who have suffered an isolated massive left ventricular infarction, this is generally not difficult for what is essentially a normal right ventricle. However, in patients who suffer nonischemic diffuse biventricular cardiomyopathy, the augmentation of preload returning to the right ventricle after implantation of an LVAD may unmask right ventricular dysfunction. In addition, under ideal circumstances right ventricular afterload should decrease, with a drop in passive pulmonary hypertension. This, however, is not always the case.

Bleeding requiring massive blood product resuscitation, hypercarbia or acidemia, mechanical pulmonary problems, and pulmonary endothelial dysfunction after cardiopulmonary bypass can increase PVR acutely after LVAD implantation. In a situation where a diseased right ventricle is already being asked to perform volume work, the imposition of pressure work in addition can be simply overwhelming. The right ventricle can perform volume work, or it can perform pressure work; but it is very rare that a right ventricle can perform both pressure and volume work simultaneously.

Finally, right ventricular developed pressure is determined by performance of the free wall of the right ventricle, as well as by position and function of the interventricular septum. As continuous-flow devices become more commonplace, an understanding of the role of the position of the interventricular septum is very important. As a continuous-flow LVAD is actuated and as the left ventricle is unloaded, the septum is "sucked" toward the left, resulting in an immediate increase in the diastolic compliance of the right ventricle. As capacitance of this chamber increases and septal contribution to right ventricular performance is taken away by suctioning it into the left ventricle, fatigue of the right ventricular free wall can occur over the next few hours, resulting in right ventricular failure. An analogy that is somewhat applicable here is that of a "hammer on an anvil," with the free wall serving as the hammer and the septum as the anvil. Increasing the distance between the hammer and the anvil requires expenditure of greater energy to deliver the blow of the hammer into the anvil. Eventually, in a diseased right ventricle, that energy requirement proves prohibitively high. The other, and more dangerous circumstance is one in which the left ventricle is allowed to distend by having pump speeds that are too low. This situation can cause immediate failure of the right ventricle by causing septal shift into the right ventricle, and immediate distension of the right ventricle.

MANAGEMENT OF RIGHT VENTRICULAR DYSFUNCTION

Meticulous attention to the conduct of the operation can enable even a patient with marginal right ventricular function to tolerate LVAD implantation, whereas sloppy technique can endanger even a well-prepared and relatively healthy right ventricle.

Patients with ischemic cardiomyopathy who have flow-limiting lesions in the right coronary artery, posterior descending coronary artery, or left anterior descending coronary artery should be revascularized at the time of LVAD implantation to salvage hibernating myocardium, and to perfuse the right ventricle and interventricular septum.

Bleeding needs to be avoided or minimized. In patients with long-standing right ventricular dysfunction and passive hepatic congestion, the synthetic function of the liver is often compromised. Accordingly, the authors pretreat patients with vitamin K on the day before operation, on the day of the operation, and postoperatively if possible. The cardiopulmonary bypass circuit is primed with fresh frozen plasma instead of crystalloid. The operative technique needs to be meticulous, with compulsive attention to hemostasis "on the way in," with particular attention to drying up the pump pocket and any sites of adhesions within the mediastinum prior to heparinization. Internalization of the LVAD is performed before heparinization to avoid driveline hematomas that can go on to become infected. The authors use Bovie electrocautery, an argon beam coagulator, and adjunctive hemostatic agents liberally.

In the rare event that the patient develops a profound coagulopathy during a particularly long, difficult, or tedious reoperative dissection, the authors pack the mediastinum with sponges and return the patient to the intensive care unit, where a blood product resuscitation is undertaken in an attempt to reverse the coagulopathy. Once corrected, the patient is returned to the operating room to proceed with LVAD implantation. If a severe coagulopathy occurs after implantation of the LVAD, a balance has to be struck between correction of the coagulopathy by blood product resuscitation and overwhelming the right ventricle by aggressively volume-loading it. In select cases, the authors may choose to pack to mediastinum and leave the chest open for 24 or 48 hours, permitting a gradual resuscitation, and then return to the operating room for a washout and chest closure. In addition, massive transfusions can result in transfusion-associated lung injury with attendant increases in PVR, which can then in turn impose pressure work on an already volume-overloaded right ventricle. The authors avoid the use of recombinant factor VII because of its prohibitive cost, as well as unpredictability and fear of thrombotic events in the setting of a freshly implanted blood–artificial surface interface.

The authors pay assiduous attention to ventilation and maintenance of the acid-base balance. Hypercarbia and acidemia can cause an increase in PVR, which can be detrimental to the performance of the right ventricle. After separating from cardiopulmonary bypass, patients are maintained on an intensive care unit ventilator both in the operating room and during transport to the intensive care unit, in an attempt to avoid perturbations in ventilatory parameters.

Although there are centers that use inhaled nitric oxide (iNO) liberally, the authors' institutional bias has been to use iNO more selectively, primarily because of its prohibitive cost. In general, iNO is used in the setting of recalcitrant right ventricular dysfunction in patients for whom right ventricular

mechanical support is not an option (eg, destination therapy patients). Alternatively, if pulmonary vascular resistance cannot be decreased by augmenting LVAD support (in the case of severe right ventricular dysfunction), the temporary addition of iNO may be used to decrease right ventricular afterload, thereby enabling more efficient use of the LVAD in the immediate postoperative period.

The authors avoid the extended use of cardiopulmonary bypass and attempt to perform the aortic anastomosis off pump, if possible, thus limiting the use of cardiopulmonary bypass (CPB) to opening the apex of the heart. In selective cases, particularly with access to the axial flow pumps and centrifugal pumps, the authors will attempt to perform the entire implantation off pump, or at the very least to continue ventilating at low tidal volumes.

Several investigators have demonstrated, over the course of the past decade, that interrupting pulmonary blood flow during CPB impairs endothelial cell signal transduction in the pulmonary arteries and branch vessels,[22] and impedes the ability of the pulmonary vasculature to relax normally, which then adversely affects right ventricular performance by imposing the requirement to do both pressure and volume work. Therefore, the authors routinely maintain ventilation despite the initiation of full CPB.

Finally, the conduct by which the patient is separated from CPB is a critically important phase of the operation. Deairing maneuvers are of critical importance. The authors routinely flood the operative field with carbon dioxide and do not initiate LVAD support until the systemic chambers are completely and thoroughly deaired, using intraoperative transesophageal echocardiography as a guide.

After actuation of the device at low flow, separation from cardiopulmonary bypass is performed very gradually, keeping a close eye on right ventricular performance. Any hemodynamic or visual sign of impeding failure (such as inability to fill the reservoir of a displacement-style pulsatile device, elevation in CVP, or sudden distension) should be met by immediate return to full CPB, reevaluation, and optimization of medical therapy. Most investigators will gradually come up to flow that can partially support the left-sided systemic circulation (ie, 3 L/min) while maintaining low flow on full CPB (ie, 2 L/min). This strategy will provide 5 L of systemic flow while forcing the right ventricle to perform only 3 L of work (while 2 L are provided by the heart lung machine). This flow can gradually be weaned, allowing the right ventricle to slowly assume its full workload.

Other investigators[23] have advocated cannulating the main pulmonary artery with a "Y" connector from the aortic line, and to separate from bypass by coming up to full flow on the LVAD, simultaneously clamping the aortic line and diverting 5 L of flow from the right atrium to the pulmonary artery, thereby providing full right heart bypass. This flow can then also be gradually weaned, allowing the right ventricle to assume its full workload. With the advent of continuous-flow devices, in which septal position is of critical importance in enabling right ventricular performance, such a strategy may hold limited appeal.

The authors pay particular attention to separating from CPB in sinus rhythm, or attempt to maintain atrioventricular synchrony with the use of temporary epicardial pacing leads. If the patient has biventricular pacing systems in place, an attempt is made to separate using these devices.

Separation from CPB is done at high, or above normal, blood pressure to maintain adequate coronary perfusion pressure. In a patient with coronary artery disease or a graft-dependent coronary circulation, particularly with volume-related distension of the right ventricle, hypotension can result in a very rapid and tight downward spiral that is very difficult to break without institution of right-sided ventricular support.

As already referred to, every effort is made to decrease right ventricular afterload with the use of intravenous phosphodiesterase inhibitors such as milrinone, along with low-dose epinephrine to promote bronchodilatation and vasodilatation of the pulmonary vasculature. In addition, as already mentioned, assiduous maintenance of the acid-base balance as well as prevention of hypercarbia and acidemia are very important. The authors also make every effort to drain pleural effusions and to treat mucus plugging or lobar collapse aggressively, and if pulmonary compliance is low will have a very low threshold to leave the chest open.

MECHANICAL CIRCULATORY SUPPORT USE: INDICATIONS FOR BIVENTRICULAR SUPPORT, ISOLATED RIGHT VENTRICULAR SUPPORT, AND TYPES OF DEVICES

The following serves as a general series of recommendations for appropriate triage for patients in end-stage heart failure being considered for mechanical circulatory support.

A hemodynamically stable patient (Intermacs profile 2, 3, or 4) with CVP less than 15, pulmonary capillary wedge pressure (PCWP) greater than 25, on stable doses of inotropes, and without pressors may be considered for LVAD implantation.

A hemodynamically stable patient (Intermacs profile 2, 3, or 4) with CVP greater than 15 and PCWP less than 25 may be considered for a

"challenge" to the right ventricle by augmenting left-sided perfusion and venous return with implantation of an intra-aortic balloon pump. If the patient is able to mobilize fluid and diurese, if PAPs remain high and do not decrease, and if CVP does not climb further, consideration may be given to proceeding to isolated LVAD implantation. If implantation of a right ventricular assist device is required, implantation should not be delayed. Leaving the operating room with borderline LVAD flows, marginal hemodynamics, low left atrial pressure, high right atrial pressures, and high doses of inotropes and/or pressors in the anticipation of recovery usually results in a suboptimal clinical outcome. Interval return to the operating room for placement of an RVAD in such a setting is usually associated with a high mortality.

A hemodynamically unstable patient (Intermacs profile 1), any patient who is dependent on pressors, who requires ECMO or mechanical ventilation, who has an unexplained fever, adult respiratory distress syndrome, hepatic or renal dysfunction, intractable ventricular arrhythmias, or an overwhelming right ventricular infarction should be considered for implantation of temporary biventricular assist device implantation. Over time, and after having been stabilized with appropriate management, some of these patients may become eligible for implantation of a permanent implantable LVAD. Others may require permanent biventricular assist device implantation, or total artificial heart implantation. Certain patients with specific and unusual presentations such as giant cell myocarditis, failed cardiac allograft, pulmonary edema despite maximal medical therapy, and ischemic cardiomyopathy whereby surgery threatens the right ventricle may be candidates for a priori permanent biventricular support.

Isolated right ventricular support may be required in the setting of a hemodynamically significant right ventricular myocardial infarction, patients in the postcardiotomy condition, in patients with end-stage cor pulmonale due to primary pulmonary disease, or in patients after heart transplantation with allograft dysfunction. In these circumstances, consideration should be given to pulmonary support with concomitant extracorporeal membrane oxygenation.

REFERENCES

1. Dang NC, Topkara VK, Mercando M, et al. Right heart failure after left ventricular assist device implantation in patients with chronic congestive heart failure. J Heart Lung Transplant 2006;25:1–6.
2. Kavarana MN, Pessin-Minsley MS, Urtecho J, et al. Right ventricular dysfunction and organ failure in

left ventricular assist device recipients: a continuing problem. Ann Thorac Surg 2002;73:745–50.

3. Deng MC, Edwards LB, Hertz MI, et al. Mechanical circulatory support device database of the ISHLT: third annual report—2005. J Heart Lung Transplant 2005; 24:1182–7.

4. Schenck S, McCarthy PM, Blackstone EH, et al. Duration of inotropic support after left ventricular assist device implantation: risk factors and impact on outcome. J Thorac Cardiovasc Surg 2006;131:447–54.

5. Morgan JA, John R, Lee BJ. Is severe right ventricular failure in left ventricular assist device recipients a risk factor for unsuccessful bridging to transplant and post-transplant mortality. Ann Thorac Surg 2004;77:859–63.

6. Wang P, Ba ZF, Chaudry IH. Differential effects of ATP-MgCl$_2$ on portal and hepatic arterial blood flow after hemorrhage and resuscitation. Am J Physiol 1992; 263:G895–900.

7. Zheng F, Wang P, Chaudry IH, et al. Alterations in tissue oxygen consumption and extraction after trauma and hemorrhagic shock. Crit Care Med 2000;28:2837–42.

8. Frazier OH, Rose EA, Oz MC, et al. Multicenter clinical evaluation of the HeartMate vented electric left ventricular assist system in patients awaiting heart transplantation. J Thorac Cardiovasc Surg 2001; 122:1186–95.

9. Rossi M, Sganga G, Mazzone M, et al. Cardiopulmonary bypass in man role of the intestine in a self-limiting inflammatory response with demonstrable bacterial translocation. Ann Thorac Surg 2004;77:612–8.

10. Rietschel ET, Brade H, Holse O, et al. Bacterial endotoxin chemical constitution, biological recognition, host response, and immunological detoxification. Curr Top Microbiol Immunol 1996;216:39–81.

11. Masai T, Sawa Y, Ohtake S, et al. Hepatic dysfunction after left ventricular mechanical assist in patients with end-stage heart failure: role of inflammatory response and hepatic microcirculation. Ann Thorac Surg 2002;73(2):549–55.

12. Frazier OH, Rose EA, Macmanus Q, et al. Multicenter clinical evaluation of the HeartMate 1000 IP left ventricular assist device. Ann Thorac Surg 1992;53:1080–90.

13. Goldstein DJ, Seldomridge JA, Chen JM, et al. Use of aprotinin in LVAD recipients reduces blood loss, blood use, and perioperative mortality. Ann Thorac Surg 1995;59:1063–8.

14. Kormos RL, Borovetz HS, Armitage JM, et al. Evolving experience with mechanical circulatory support. Ann Surg 1991;214:471–7.

15. Kormos RL, Gasior TA, Kawai A, et al. Transplant candidate's clinical status rather than right ventricular function defines need for univentricular versus biventricular support. J Thorac Cardiovasc Surg 1996;111:773–83.

16. Pagani FD, Lynch W, Swaniker F, et al. Extracorporeal life support to left ventricular assist device bridge to heart transplant: A strategy to optimize survival and resource utilization. Circulation 1999; 100(Suppl 19):II206–10.

17. Fukamachi K, McCarthy PM, Smedira NG, et al. Preoperative risk factors for right ventricular failure after implantable left ventricular assist device insertion. Ann Thorac Surg 1999;68:2181–4.

18. Ochiai Y, McCarthy PM, Smerdira NG, et al. Predictors of severe right ventricular failure after implantable left ventricular assist device insertion: analysis of 245 patients. Circulation 2002;106(Suppl 1): I198–202.

19. Matthews JC, Koelling TM, Pagani FD, et al. The right ventricular failure risk score a pre-operative tool for assessing the risk of right ventricular failure in left ventricular assist device candidates. J Am Coll Cardiol 2008;51(22):2163–72.

20. Smedira NG, Massad MG, Navia J, et al. Pulmonary hypertension is not a risk factor for RVAD use and death after left ventricular assist system support. ASAIO J 1996;42:M733–5.

21. Fararr DJ, Hill JD, Pennington DG, et al. Preoperative and postoperative comparison of patients with univentricular and biventricular support with the Thoratec ventricular assist device as a bridge to cardiac transplantation. J Thorac Cardiovasc Surg 1997;113:202–9.

22. Enisa MF. Pulmonary protection during cardiac surgery: systematic literature review. Asian Cardiovasc Thorac Ann 2008;16:503–7.

23. Loebe M, Potapov E, Sodian R, et al. A safe and simple method of preserving right ventricular function during implantation of a left ventricular assist device. J Thorac Cardiovasc Surg 2001;122:1043.

Editors' Comments on "Right Ventricular Dysfunction in Patients Undergoing Left Ventricular Assist Device Implantation: Predictors, Management and Device Utilization"

John A. Elefteriades, MD

KEY CONCEPTS

Right ventricular (RV) failure after left ventricular assist device (LVAD) placement is common and often lethal. The reader must keep the RV in mind and avoid left ventricle "tunnel vision."

STRENGTHS

In "Right Ventricular Dysfunction in Patients Undergoing Left Ventricular Assist Device Implantation: Predictors, Management and Device Utilization," Dr Abeel Mangi reviews comprehensively how to predict vulnerability to RV failure after LVAD, how to prevent this, and how and when to institute mechanical RV support. In terms of clinical parameters, hemodynamic instability and renal and hepatic dysfunction indicate that RV failure is likely. In terms of hemodynamic parameters, low cardiac output, high central venous pressure, and low pulmonary artery pressures (indicating a weak RV unable to generate pressure) predict that RV failure is likely. On echocardiography, loss of the normal triangular RV shape, with assumption of a globular morphology; RV hypocontractility; and tricuspid insufficiency all are indicators of a precarious right-sided situation likely to result in RV failure after LVAD. Support is provided for the age-old cardiac surgical adage "If you even think you may need to use RV mechanical support, do it; if you don't, later will be too late."

WEAKNESSES

Despite considerable scientific clarification of the pathophysiology, clinical predictors, and optimal medical and mechanical treatments of RV failure after LVAD, investigators are far from solving this problem or preventing its powerful adverse impact on pretransplant and posttransplant survival.

Section of Cardiac Surgery, Yale University School of Medicine, Boardman 2, 333 Cedar Street, New Haven, CT 06510, USA
E-mail address: john.elefteriades@yale.edu

Cardiol Clin 29 (2011) 639
doi:10.1016/j.ccl.2011.07.009
0733-8651/11/$ – see front matter © 2011 Published by Elsevier Inc.

Can the Occurrence of Gastrointestinal Bleeding in Nonpulsatile Left Ventricular Assist Device Patients Provide Clues for the Reversal of Arteriosclerosis?

Louis H. Stein, MD, John A. Elefteriades, MD*

KEYWORDS
- Gastrointestinal bleeding • Arteriosclerosis
- Left ventricular assist devices • von Willebrand factor

Continuous-flow left ventricular assist devices (CF-LVADs) such as the (Jarvik 2000, Jarvik Heart, New York, NY, USA), the (Incor, Berlin, Germany), and the (HeartMate II, Thoratec Corporation, Pleasanton, CA, USA) have become fixtures in the armamentarium for treatment of end-stage heart disease.[1,2] The HeartMate II has demonstrated its efficacy in circulatory support up for up to 2 years.[3] CF-LVADs, in combination with pharmacotherapy, have been demonstrated to be useful in bridge-to-recovery treatment in patients with nonischemic cardiomyopathy.[4] Furthermore, these devices are associated with improvements in patient functional status and quality of life.[2] The more compact design of CF-LVADs facilitates their implantation, with less tissue dissection and less bulk of implanted material.

CONCERNS ABOUT ORGAN FUNCTION WITH NONPULSATILE FLOW: RELIEVED

Initially, these devices were met with some trepidation, as concerns were raised that the nonpulsatile flow they deliver may have deleterious effects on end-organ function. After all, the natural circulatory state is a pulsatile one. It is certainly un-nerving for a patient to present to emergency room or clinic—conscious, looking and feeling well, but with no pulse. Clinical data, however, did not support this concern. Kidney function, measured by serum creatinine (CS), and liver function, measured total bilirubin, aspartate aminotransferase (AST), and serum glutamic pyruvic transaminase (SGPT), were maintained or improved in a cohort of 10 patients supported with a Jarvik 2000.[5] In their survey of 309 patients supported

Section of Cardiac Surgery, Yale University School of Medicine, Boardman 2, 333 Cedar Street, New Haven, CT 06510, USA
* Corresponding author.
E-mail address: john.elefteriades@yale.edu

Cardiol Clin 29 (2011) 641–645
doi:10.1016/j.ccl.2011.08.010
0733-8651/11/$ – see front matter © 2011 Elsevier Inc. All rights reserved.

with the Heartmate II device, a persistent improvement in AST, alanine aminostransferase (ALT), serum urea nitrogen, and Cr was observed up to 6 months.[6] Patients supported with pulsatile and CF-LVADs demonstrated similar improvement in these end-organ indicies.[7,8]

CHANGES IN VASCULAR BIOLOGY WITH NONPULSATILE FLOW
Changes in Hemostatic Mechanisms

In spite of these encouraging results, some surprising trends have been identified, which may indicate fundamental alterations in vascular endothelial physiology in the setting of—and possibly as a direct consequence of—nonpulsatile flow.

Several studies have reported a propensity for gastrointestinal (GI) bleeding in patients supported with CF-LVAD.[9–11] See **Fig. 1**. These episodes occur in patients without a prior history of GI bleeding[10] and do not appear to occur in patients with pulsatile support devices.[11] The mechanism of this phenomenon remains to be elucidated. Because of its rarity, large studies of these GI bleeding events are practically impossible. Bleeding after nonpulsatile LVAD placement seems to be due predominantly to intestinal arteriovenous malformations (AVMs) (see **Fig. 2**). These are thin walled vessels with endothelium and adventitia, but little media—accounting for the very thin wall. Interestingly, bleeding tends to disappear when cardiac transplantation is performed, the LVAD removed, and pulsatile blood flow restored. Some authors have noted a parallel between the GI bleeding with nonpulsatile LVAD support and the propensity

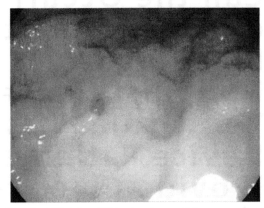

Fig. 2. Multiple AVMs in the gastric mucosa of a patient maintained on long-term nonpulsatile left ventricular assist device support. (*From* Demirozu ZT, Radovancevic R, Hochman LF, et al. Arteriovenous malformation and gastrointestinal bleeding in patients with the HeartMate II left ventricular assist device. J Heart Lung Transp 2011;30:849–53; with permission.)

toward GI bleeding seen in patients with aortic stenosis, the latter of which has been given the eponym Heyde syndrome.[10,12] This GI bleeding related to aortic stenosis also frequently arises in AVMs, and the etiology of the link between the valvular disease and the vascular malformations remains obscure. This similarity has driven many of the investigations of the mechanism of GI bleeding in patients supported with CF-LVAD.

An acquired type 2A von Willebrand syndrome has been implicated in GI bleeding seen with aortic stenosis.[13] This has been attributed to increased proteolysis of high molecular weight (HMW) components of vWF (von Willebrand factor) from increased shear forces in aortic stenosis.[14] vWF levels improve in aortic stenosis patients following aortic valve replacement.[15,16] A similar decrease in the level of vWF protein has been demonstrated in patients with CF-LVAD.[17,18] Conversely, vWF levels have been found to normalize after axial flow device explantation.[19] Interestingly, one case report demonstrates an acquired vWF deficiency after a HeartMate XVE (pulsatile) was exchanged for a HeartMate II (nonpulsatile).[20] Thus in both aortic stenosis and CF-LVADs, increased shear forces induce the proteolysis of HMW components of vWF, resulting in a tendency toward bleeding.

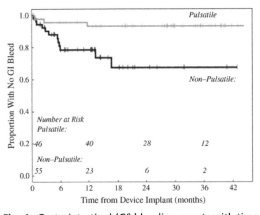

Fig. 1. Gastrointestinal (*GI*) bleeding events with time after left ventricular assist device placement in 101 patients. (*Reproduced from* Crow S, John R, Boyle A, et al. Gastrointestinal bleeding rates in recipients of nonpulsatile and pulsatile left ventricular assist devices. J Thorac Cardiovasc Surg 2009;137(1):211; with permission.)

Changes in Vascular Physiology and Morphology

It has also been noted that in aortic stenosis, there is a dampening of pulse pressure resulting in a blunted arterial waveform and a less pulsatile flow pattern that may be similar to a CF-LVAD. It

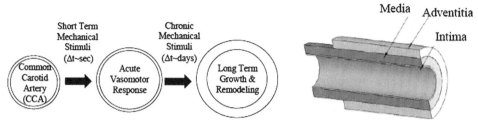

Fig. 3. Schematic representation of remodeling (thickening) of arterial wall (especially the media) in response to mechanical stimulation of pulsatile flow. The authors speculate that this process can be reversed with institution of nonpulsatile flow during left ventricular assist device support. (*From* Eberth JF. Arterial biomechanics and the influence of pulsatility on growth and remodeling. PhD dissertation. Bioengineering. Texas A & M University; 2008; with permission.)

is clear that changes in the rheology of blood flow affect the physiology of arterial endothelium, with consequent changes in arterial structure. Yao and colleagues identified changes in arterial remodeling due to alterations in pulsatility using an ex vivo model.[21] Their study found fenestrae size decreased in both hyperpulsatile and nonpulsatile arteries, while collagen 1 and connexin 43 expression increased only in arteries with hyperpulsatile flow.[21] Thus, they found that "climination [of] pulse pressure from its normal physiologic level stimulates arterial wall matrix structure changes." Similarly, atherosclerosis is associated with increased tissue factor expression, which is increased with pulsatile flow.[22] Rossi and colleagues investigated the relationship between the effect of flow pattern (steady, nonreversing pulsatile, and oscillating), statin concentration, and human aortic endothelial cell mRNA expression.[23] Their data indicate that Kruppel-like factor 2 (KLF2), endothelial nitric oxide synthase (eNOS), and thrombomodulin (TM) expression were upregulated by statins, steady flow and nonreversing pulsatile flow.[23] Furthermore, oscillating flow decreased the endothelial cell's responsiveness to statins.

Pulse pressure per se has been identified as an independent risk factor for development of arterial stiffening and arteriosclerotic vascular disease (PVD).[21,24] Ascending aortic pulse pressure has been associated with coronary atherosclerosis[25,26] and with restenosis after coronary artery angioplasty.[27,28] Interestingly, increased ascending aortic pulse pressure has also been related to occlusion of sapheous vein grafts used in coronary bypass surgery.[29] This arteriosclerosis, of course, is manifested grossly as thickening of the arterial vessel wall (see **Fig. 3**).

The converse has also been noted anecdotally by surgeons. That is, that arteries (aorta, femorals) exposed long-term to the nonpulsatility of CF-LVADs tend to be thinner—in fact, vein-like—in their gross morphology (personal observation: J. Elefteriades, MD). That is, gross observation has shown that nonpulsatile flow tends to render arteries more thin-walled over time—as if the body senses the decreased pressure load and wall stress and reacts adaptively by allowing the arterial wall to become thinner, like a low-pressure vein. It has been known for decades, and recently demonstrated experimentally, that the pulmonary artery undergoes involution and wall thinning when perfused in a nonpulsatile function, coming to resemble a vein rather than an artery.[30] Recent evidence also indicates that even

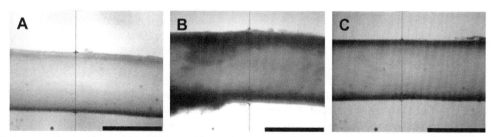

Fig. 4. Images of carotid arteries within a mechanical testing device. (*A*) baseline, (*B*) subjected to high pulsatile conditions, and (*C*) subjected to low pulsatile conditions. Figures are to scale, and the black bar represents 660 μg. (*From* Eberth JF. Arterial biomechanics and the influence of pulsatility on growth and remodeling. PhD dissertation. Bioengineering. Texas A & M University; 2008; with permission.)

in utero, pulsatility is essential for arterial rather than venous identity of developing blood vessels.[31] Additional recent experimental evidence confirms that arterial morphology and thickness is plastic, depending on the degree of pulse pressure.[32] The arterial wall does become thinner and somewhat atrophic under the influence of nonpulsatile flow in experimental animals[33–36] (see **Fig. 4**). This article is written not only to explore the deleterious effects of nonpulsatile flow (namely, GI bleeding), but also to propose the novel concept that deliberate induction of nonpulsatile flow might be harnessed to produce beneficial remodeling in arteriosclerotic arteries.

SUMMARY

CF-LVADs have proven their efficacy in the treatment of end-stage heart disease. They are a reliable option in bridge-to-transplant and destination therapy. An enigmatic consequence of this therapy has been occult GI bleeding. A clear component of this phenomenon has been perturbation of vWF levels, although other factors likely contribute. The authors believe that decreased pulsatility results in changes in cellular protein expression and ultimately vascular morphology. This could further explain the GI bleeding seen in patients supported with axial flow devices and with aortic stenosis—on the basis of arteriovenous-like thinning of small-caliber intestinal vessels. Further, the authors hypothesize that axial flow may possibly be applied in the future deliberately to stimulate beneficial remodeling of coronary arteries (or other arterial vessels) affected by atherosclerosis. Could such beneficial remodeling also potentiate bridge to recovery? More study is required to identify the effects of long-term axial flow support on vascular phenotype, but the possibility is raised that it may be possible to delay or reverse arteriosclerosis by harnessing beneficially an unanticipated side effect of nonpulsatile flow–thinning of the arterial wall as a consequence of decreased wall stress.

REFERENCES

1. Miller LW, Pagani FD, Russell SD, et al. Use of a continuous-flow device in patients awaiting heart transplantation. N Engl J Med 2007;357(9):885–96.
2. Pagani FD, Miller LW, Russell SD, et al. Extended mechanical circulatory support with a continuous-flow rotary left ventricular assist device. J Am Coll Cardiol 2009;54(4):312–21.
3. Slaughter MS, Rogers JG, Milano CA, et al. Advanced heart failure treated with continuous-flow left ventricular assist device. N Engl J Med 2009; 361(23):2241–51.
4. Birks EJ, George RS, Hedger M, et al. Reversal of severe heart failure with a continuous-flow left ventricular assist device and pharmacological therapy: a prospective study. Circulation 2011;123(4):381–90.
5. Letsou GV, Myers TJ, Gregoric ID, et al. Continuous axial-flow left ventricular assist device (Jarvik 2000) maintains kidney and liver perfusion for up to 6 months. Ann Thorac Surg 2003;76(4):1167–70.
6. Russell SD, Rogers JG, Milano CA, et al. Renal and hepatic function improve in advanced heart failure patients during continuous-flow support with the HeartMate II left ventricular assist device. Circulation 2009;120(23):2352–7.
7. Radovancevic B, Vrtovec B, de Kort E, et al. End-organ function in patients on long-term circulatory support with continuous- or pulsatile-flow assist devices. J Heart Lung Transplant 2007;26(8): 815–8.
8. Kamdar F, Boyle A, Liao K, et al. Effects of centrifugal, axial, and pulsatile left ventricular assist device support on end-organ function in heart failure patients. J Heart Lung Transplant 2009;28(4):352–9.
9. Stern DR, Kazam J, Edwards P, et al. Increased incidence of gastrointestinal bleeding following implantation of the HeartMate II LVAD. J Card Surg 2010; 25(3):352–6.
10. Letsou GV, Shah N, Gregoric ID, et al. Gastrointestinal bleeding from arteriovenous malformations in patients supported by the Jarvik 2000 axial-flow left ventricular assist device. J Heart Lung Transplant 2005;24(1):105–9.
11. Crow S, John R, Boyle A, et al. Gastrointestinal bleeding rates in recipients of nonpulsatile and pulsatile left ventricular assist devices. J Thorac Cardiovasc Surg 2009;137(1):208–15.
12. Heyde EC. Gastrointestinal bleeding in aortic stenosis. N Engl J Med 1958;259:196.
13. Vincentelli A, Susen S, Le Tourneau T, et al. Acquired von Willebrand syndrome in aortic stenosis. N Engl J Med 2003;349(4):343–9.
14. Pareti FI, Lattuada A, Bressi C, et al. Proteolysis of von Willebrand factor and shear stress-induced platelet aggregation in patients with aortic valve stenosis. Circulation 2000;102(11):1290–5.
15. Morishima A, Marui A, Shimamoto T, et al. Successful aortic valve replacement for Heyde syndrome with confirmed hematologic recovery. Ann Thorac Surg 2007;83(1):287–8.
16. Gola W, Lelonek M. Clinical implication of gastrointestinal bleeding in degenerative aortic stenosis: an update. Cardiol J 2010;17(4):330–4.
17. Crow S, Chen D, Milano C, et al. Acquired von Willebrand syndrome in continuous-flow ventricular assist device recipients. Ann Thorac Surg 2010; 90(4):1263–9 [discussion: 1269].

18. Crow S, Milano C, Joyce L, et al. Comparative analysis of von Willebrand factor profiles in pulsatile and continuous left ventricular assist device recipients. ASAIO J 2010;56(5):441–5.

19. Meyer AL, Malehsa D, Bara C, et al. Acquired von Willebrand syndrome in patients with an axial flow left ventricular assist device. Circ Heart Fail 2010; 3(6):675–81.

20. Malehsa D, Meyer AL, Bara C, et al. Acquired von Willebrand syndrome after exchange of the Heart-Mate XVE to the HeartMate II ventricular assist device. Eur J Cardiothorac Surg 2009;35(6):1091–3.

21. Yao Q, Hayman DM, Dai Q, et al. Alterations of pulse pressure stimulate arterial wall matrix remodeling. J Biomech Eng 2009;131(10):101011.

22. Abe R, Yamashita N, Rochier A, et al. Pulsatile to-fro flow induces greater and sustained expression of tissue factor RNA in HUVEC than unidirectional laminar flow. Am J Physiol Heart Circ Physiol 2011; 300(4):H1345–51.

23. Rossi J, Jonak P, Rouleau L, et al. Differential response of endothelial cells to simvastatin when conditioned with steady, nonreversing pulsatile or oscillating shear stress. Ann Biomed Eng 2011; 39(1):402–13.

24. Safar ME. Pulse pressure, arterial stiffness and wave reflections (augmentation index) as cardiovascular risk factors in hypertension. Ther Adv Cardiovasc Dis 2008;2(1):13–24.

25. Mourad JJ, Danchin N, Rudnichi A, et al. Aortic pulse pressure and atherosclerotic structural alterations of coronary arteries. J Hum Hypertens 2010; 24(1):51–7.

26. Guray Y, Guray U, Altay H, et al. Aortic pulse pressure and aortic pulsatility are associated with angiographic coronary artery disease in women. Blood Press 2005;14(5):293–7.

27. Lu TM, Hsu NW, Chen YH, et al. Pulsatility of ascending aorta and restenosis after coronary angioplasty in patients >60 years of age with stable angina pectoris. Am J Cardiol 2001;88(9): 964–8.

28. Nakayama Y, Tsumura K, Yamashita N, et al. Pulsatility of ascending aortic pressure waveform is a powerful predictor of restenosis after percutaneous transluminal coronary angioplasty. Circulation 2000;101(5):470–2.

29. Cay S, Cagirci G, Balbay Y, et al. Effect of aortic pulse and fractional pulse pressures on early patency of sapheneous vein grafts. Coron Artery Dis 2008;19(7):435–9.

30. Zongtao Y, Huishan W, Zengwei W, et al. Experimental study of nonpulsatile flow perfusion and structural remodeling of pulmonary microcirculation vessels. Thorac Cardiovasc Surg 2010;58(8):468–72.

31. Buschmann I, Pries A, Styp-Rekowska B, et al. Pulsatile shear and Gja5 modulate arterial identity and remodeling events during flow-driven arteriogenesis. Development 2010;137:2187–96.

32. Eberth JF. Arterial biomechanics and the influence of pulsatility on growth and remodeling. PhD dissertation. Bioengineering. Texas A & M University; 2008.

33. Thalmann M, Schima H, Wieselthaler G, et al. Physiology of continuous blood flow in recipients of rotary cardiac assist devices. J Heart Lung Transplant 2005;24:237–45.

34. Nishimura T, Tatsumi E, Taenaka Y, et al. Effects of long-term nonpulsatile left heart bypass on the mechanical properties of the aortic wall. ASAIO J 1999;45:455–9.

35. Nishimura T, Tatsumi E, Nishinaka T, et al. Prolonged nonpulsatile left heart bypass diminishes vascular contractility. Int J Artif Organs 1999;22:492–8.

36. Nishimura T, Tatsumi E, Nishinaka T, et al. Diminished vasoconstrictive function caused by long-term non-pulsatile left heart bypass. Artif Organs 1999;23:722–6.

Editorial Comment on "Can the Occurrence of GI Bleeding in Non-Pulsatile LVAD Patients Provide Clues for the Reversal of Arteriosclerosis?"

John A. Elefteriades, MD

KEY CONCEPTS

The authors of "Can the Occurrence of GI Bleeding in Non-Pulsatile LVAD Patients Provide Clues for the Reversal of Arteriosclerosis?" (Drs John A. Elefteriades and Louis H. Stein) make the point that arterial morphology is highly dependent on mechanical loading, especially the pulse pressure of the arterial waveform. With nonpulsatile flow of axial LVADs, the mechanical loading is light and the arterial wall involutes, thinning and losing smooth muscle cells. This observation may provide a mechanism for stopping or reversing arteriosclerosis via LVAD therapy in the future.

STRENGTHS

The dependence of arterial morphology on mechanical loading conditions is well demonstrated. The concept of deliberately manipulating this dependence via LVAD therapy is novel.

WEAKNESSES

The potential for therapy for arteriosclerosis via this means is at present speculative.

Section of Cardiac Surgery, Yale University School of Medicine, Boardman 2, 333 Cedar Street, New Haven, CT 06510, USA
E-mail address: john.elefteriades@yale.edu

Cardiol Clin 29 (2011) 647
doi:10.1016/j.ccl.2011.07.002
0733-8651/11/$ – see front matter © 2011 Published by Elsevier Inc.

Editorial Comment on "Can the Occurrence of GI Bleeding in Non-Pulsatile LVAD Patients Provide Clues for the Reversal of Arteriosclerosis?"

Index

Note: Page numbers of article titles are in **boldface** type.

Cardiol Clin 29 (2011) 649–654
doi:10.1016/S0733-8651(11)00104-4
0733-8651/11/$ – see front matter © 2011 Elsevier Inc. All rights reserved.

cardiology.theclinics.com

United States Postal Service

Statement of Ownership, Management, and Circulation
(All Periodicals Publications Except Requestor Publications)

1. Publication Title	2. Publication Number	3. Filing Date
Cardiology Clinics	0 0 0 - 7 0 1	9/16/11

4. Issue Frequency	5. Number of Issues Published Annually	6. Annual Subscription Price
Feb, May, Aug, Nov	4	$282.00

7. Complete Mailing Address of Known Office of Publication (Not printer) (Street, city, county, state, and ZIP+4®)

Elsevier Inc.
360 Park Avenue South
New York, NY 10010-1710

Contact Person: Amy S. Beacham
Telephone (Include area code): 215-239-3687

8. Complete Mailing Address of Headquarters or General Business Office of Publisher (Not printer)

Elsevier Inc., 360 Park Avenue South, New York, NY 10010-1710

9. Full Names and Complete Mailing Addresses of Publisher, Editor, and Managing Editor (Do not leave blank)

Publisher (Name and complete mailing address)

Kim Murphy, Elsevier, Inc., 1600 John F. Kennedy Blvd. Suite 1800, Philadelphia, PA 19103-2899

Editor (Name and complete mailing address)

Barbara Cohen-Kligerman, Elsevier, Inc., 1600 John F. Kennedy Blvd. Suite 1800, Philadelphia, PA 19103-2899

Managing Editor (Name and complete mailing address)

Barbara Cohen-Kligerman, Elsevier, Inc., 1600 John F. Kennedy Blvd. Suite 1800, Philadelphia, PA 19103-2899

10. Owner (Do not leave blank. If the publication is owned by a corporation, give the name and address of the corporation immediately followed by the names and addresses of all stockholders owning or holding 1 percent or more of the total amount of stock. If not owned by a corporation, give the names and addresses of the individual owners. If owned by a partnership or other unincorporated firm, give its name and address as well as those of each individual owner. If the publication is published by a nonprofit organization, give its name and address.)

Full Name	Complete Mailing Address
Wholly owned subsidiary of	4520 East-West Highway
Reed/Elsevier, US holdings	Bethesda, MD 20814

11. Known Bondholders, Mortgagees, and Other Security Holders Owning or Holding 1 Percent or More of Total Amount of Bonds, Mortgages, or Other Securities. If none, check box. ☐ None

Full Name	Complete Mailing Address
N/A	

12. Tax Status (For completion by nonprofit organizations authorized to mail at nonprofit rates) (Check one)
The purpose, function, and nonprofit status of this organization and the exempt status for federal income tax purposes:
☐ Has Not Changed During Preceding 12 Months
☐ Has Changed During Preceding 12 Months (Publisher must submit explanation of change with this statement)

PS Form 3526, September 2007 (Page 1 of 3 (Instructions Page 3)) PSN 7530-01-000-9931 PRIVACY NOTICE: See our Privacy policy in www.usps.com

---

13. Publication Title	14. Issue Date for Circulation Data Below
Cardiology Clinics	August 2011

15. Extent and Nature of Circulation		Average No. Copies Each Issue During Preceding 12 Months	No. Copies of Single Issue Published Nearest to Filing Date
a. Total Number of Copies (Net press run)		1614	1675
b. Paid Circulation (By Mail and Outside the Mail)	(1) Mailed Outside-County Paid Subscriptions Stated on PS Form 3541. (Include paid distribution above nominal rate, advertiser's proof copies, and exchange copies)	529	485
	(2) Mailed In-County Paid Subscriptions Stated on PS Form 3541 (Include paid distribution above nominal rate, advertiser's proof copies, and exchange copies)		
	(3) Paid Distribution Outside the Mails Including Sales Through Dealers and Carriers, Street Vendors, Counter Sales, and Other Paid Distribution Outside USPS®	235	233
	(4) Paid Distribution by Other Classes Mailed Through the USPS (e.g. First-Class Mail®)		
c. Total Paid Distribution (Sum of 15b (1), (2), (3), and (4))	▶	764	718
d. Free or Nominal Rate Distribution (By Mail and Outside the Mail)	(1) Free or Nominal Rate Outside-County Copies Included on PS Form 3541	52	60
	(2) Free or Nominal Rate In-County Copies Included on PS Form 3541		
	(3) Free or Nominal Rate Copies Mailed at Other Classes Through the USPS (e.g. First-Class Mail)		
	(4) Free or Nominal Rate Distribution Outside the Mail (Carriers or other means)		
e. Total Free or Nominal Rate Distribution (Sum of 15d (1), (2), (3) and (4))	▶	52	60
f. Total Distribution (Sum of 15c and 15e)	▶	816	778
g. Copies not Distributed (See instructions to publishers #4 (page #3))	▶	798	897
h. Total (Sum of 15f and g)	▶	1614	1675
i. Percent Paid (15c divided by 15f times 100)		93.63%	92.29%

16. Publication of Statement of Ownership
☐ If the publication is a general publication, publication of this statement is required. Will be printed in the November 2011 issue of this publication. ☐ Publication not required.

17. Signature and Title of Editor, Publisher, Business Manager, or Owner

[signature] Amy S. Beacham – Senior Inventory Distribution Coordinator

Date: September 16, 2011

I certify that all information furnished on this form is true and complete. I understand that anyone who furnishes false or misleading information on this form or who omits material or information requested on the form may be subject to criminal sanctions (including fines and imprisonment) and/or civil sanctions (including civil penalties).

PS Form 3526, September 2007 (Page 2 of 3)

Moving?

Make sure your subscription moves with you!

To notify us of your new address, find your **Clinics Account Number** (located on your mailing label above your name), and contact customer service at:

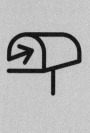

Email: journalscustomerservice-usa@elsevier.com

800-654-2452 (subscribers in the U.S. & Canada)
314-447-8871 (subscribers outside of the U.S. & Canada)

Fax number: 314-447-8029

Elsevier Health Sciences Division
Subscription Customer Service
3251 Riverport Lane
Maryland Heights, MO 63043

ELSEVIER

Printed and bound by CPI Group (UK) Ltd, Croydon, CR0 4YY

03/10/2024

01040357-0009